P9-CCO-855

THE EVERYGIRL'S
GUIDE TO DIET AND FITNESS

HOW I LOST 40 LBS AND KEPT IT OFF– AND HOW YOU CAN TOO!

MARIA MENOUNOS

WITH KEVEN UNDERGARO

ZINC INK

BALLANTINE BOOKS

New York

No book can replace the diagnostic expertise and medical advice of a trusted physician. Please be certain to consult with your doctor before making any decisions that affect your health or extreme changes to your diet, particularly if you suffer from any medical condition or have any symptom that may require treatment.

As of press time, the URLs displayed in this book link or refer to existing websites on the Internet. Penguin Random House is not responsible for, and should not be deemed to endorse or recommend, any website or content available on the Internet (including without limitation at any website, blog page, information page) other than its own.

A Zinc Ink Trade Paperback Original

Copyright © 2014 by EveryGirl's Guide, LLC

All rights reserved.

Published in the United States by Zinc Ink, an imprint of Random House, a division of Random House LLC, a Penguin Random House Company, New York.

BALLANTINE and the HOUSE colophon are registered trademarks of Random House LLC.

ZINC INK is a trademark of David Zinczenko.
The EveryGirl's Guide is a trademark of EveryGirl's Guide, LLC

ISBN 978-0-8041-7713-9

eBook ISBN 978-0-8041-7712-2

Printed in the United States of America on acid-free paper

www.ballantinebooks.com

24689753

Design by Mike Smith

Inside photography: Elise Donoghue
Cover and title page photography: Ashley Barrett

Giants Bikini photo: Neilson Barnard/Getty Images Entertainment/Getty Images
Dancing with the Stars images:
copyright Bob D'Amico/American Broadcasting Companies, Inc.
copyright Adam Taylor/American Broadcasting Companies, Inc.
Celebrity headshots and red carpet courtesy: Startraksphoto.com
Perez Hilton photos: after photo: Matt Barnes; before photo: Perez Hilton
Additional interior photography: Stephen Lemieux
Keven Undergaro headshot: Andrew Eccles/Oxygen Media
Grecian Delight photo: Randall Slavin Photography
Jack LaLanne photos courtesy: Jacklalanne.com, The LaLanne Family

"To my father, Costas. You worked three jobs and never had much free time or money, yet you were able to achieve the most important goal of diet and fitness: being healthy and productive in your later years. I love you, Dad, for this and so many other reasons and thank God every day for having you in my life. You are the inspiration for this book, and I hope what I've learned from you helps others achieve similar success."

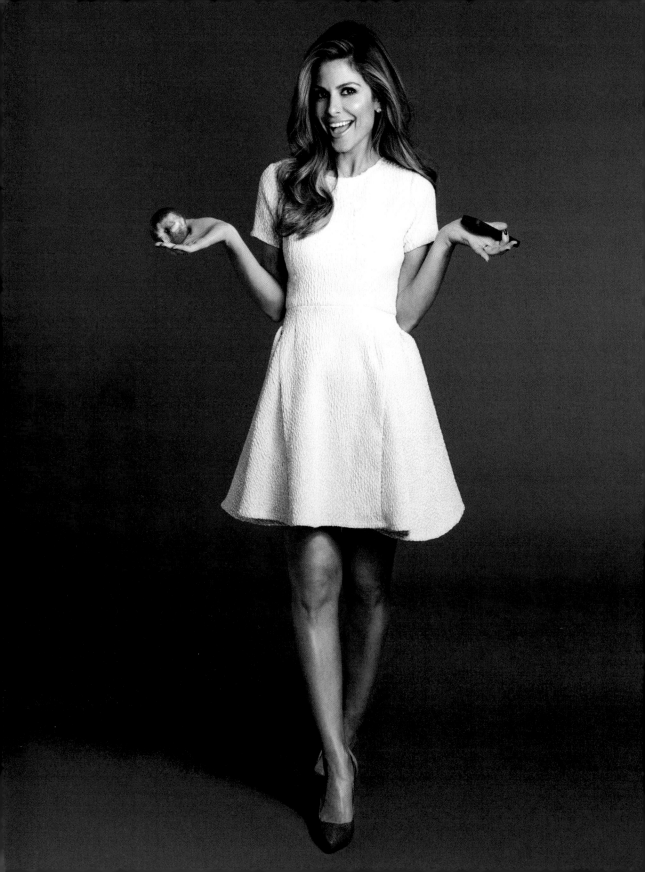

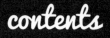

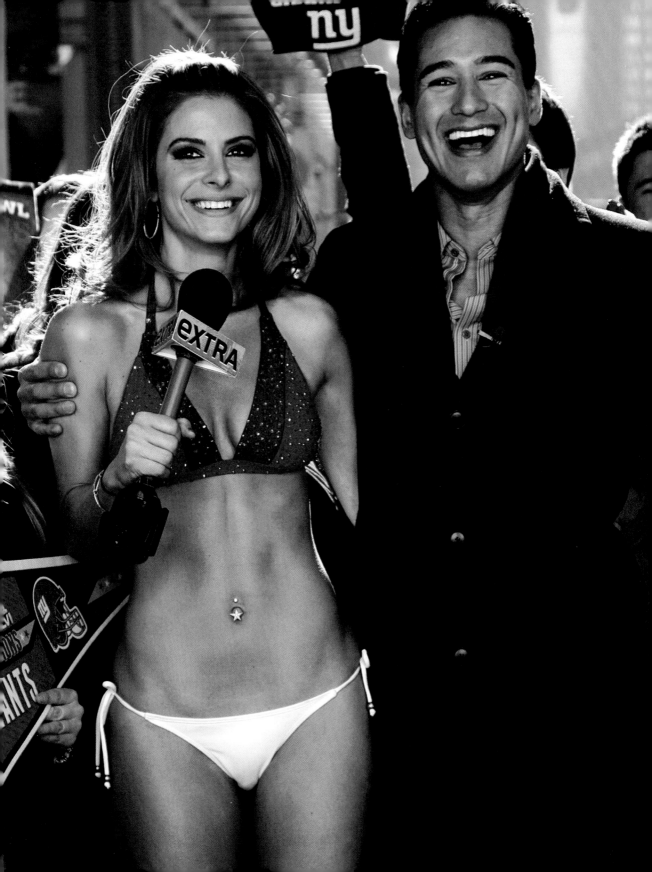

introduction

EveryGirl (n): A term in this book that literally refers to every girl out there, young or old, single or married, rich or poor who lacks time in their day and money to spend, either because they are struggling financially or are just wise and thrifty, but more than anything wants to improve their lives and to grow.

Some of you may know me from TV—hosting shows like *Extra,* competing on *Dancing with the Stars,* and wrestling for the WWE—or from seeing me in the weekly magazines. You might have even caught me posing in a bikini on the cover of health publications like *Shape* and *Self.* But what you may not know is that I was once forty pounds heavier.

I had hit 160 pounds by gaining a little weight year after year, and at 5'7½", I was dangerously close to being seriously overweight. I knew that unless I did something, there was no reason to think that I wouldn't just keep gaining. But what could I do? I had tried a ton of diets but didn't have the willpower to stay on any of them for longer than three days. I had very little time in my schedule and no money. Sound familiar?

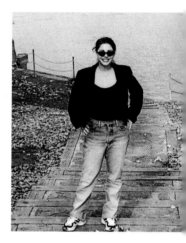

↑ Size 14. Funny enough, even at this weight and size, I had a smaller upper body and stomach. But I was a double D and had a shelf for a butt! And yes, I know, my fashion isn't what it is now.

↖ I lost a Super Bowl bet at *Extra* and was forced to host the show in a NY Giants bikini. It was mortifying and freezing!!

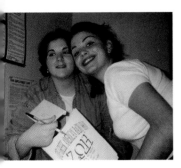

↑ With my friend Deidre working on my Greek-American radio show

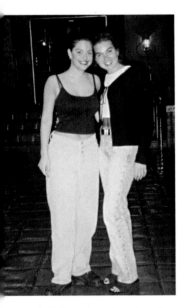

↑ Ahhh . . . the college days. Here with a college bud, Tiffany, on my first trip to L.A. Size 12 here.

Just like many of you, I was an EveryGirl—someone who had worked hard and wanted to be healthy and successful, but had to accomplish it all on her own and with limited resources. So relying on the way I was raised, some common sense, and much trial and error, I came up with a plan not only to lose the weight, but also, many years later, to keep it off. It worked—and more important, it keeps working!

I still consider myself an EveryGirl. When it comes to my weight and health, even though I'm on TV, I have many of the same obstacles I've always had. I'm still busy, I still have a family history of health problems (more on that later), and I am still careful with money. Obviously, I can't fall back on having "good genes"—that's what packed on those extra forty pounds to begin with!—so I have to make healthy eating and fitness a priority and put in the work.

At the same time, however, I still eat stuff like loaded potato skins and nachos. And guess what: There are times when I gain a few pounds here and there, too. I've just found simple, practical, and affordable ways to balance my diet and exercise routine with the occasional indulgence in order to return to my desired weight.

I don't have an official daily diet or workout plan. What I do have is a lifestyle plan that every girl of every background and age can follow. Yes, my plan will help you lose weight and get in shape, but the real key is that it will help you to live a longer, healthier, and more prosperous life. You don't need a lot of money, and you don't need a lot of time—the very things every girl seems to lack most today. You don't even need to have a lot of willpower or do a lot of work when you compare my approach to most structured diet and exercise plans. You mainly need patience and an open mind to the possibilities.

THE EVERYGIRL'S GUIDE TO DIET AND FITNESS

Throughout the book I've included several interviews with celebrity friends and experts. Some of their advice may strike a chord that will help you on your path to a healthier, fitter life. Over the past fourteen years, I've had the opportunity to interview leading trainers, dietitians, and researchers. Even though the strategies I used to drop the forty pounds are still the same techniques I swear by today, I've kept an open mind and used what I have learned from these experts to fine-tune my approach. This book is my opportunity to share all of that knowledge with you.

Ultimately, the idea is for you to be armed with enough information to get you on the right path and keep you there. And, of course, while I hope this book helps you lose weight, my sincerest hope is that it gets you focused on the greater goal: to live a long and healthy life!

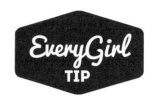

TAB NOW, REREAD LATER

Keep sticky notes or tabs handy while reading this book. Women come up to me all the time holding my last book all marked up with tabs. I think it's a great idea and want to share it with you. Highlight anything you may want to add to your information bank or inspiration boards later.

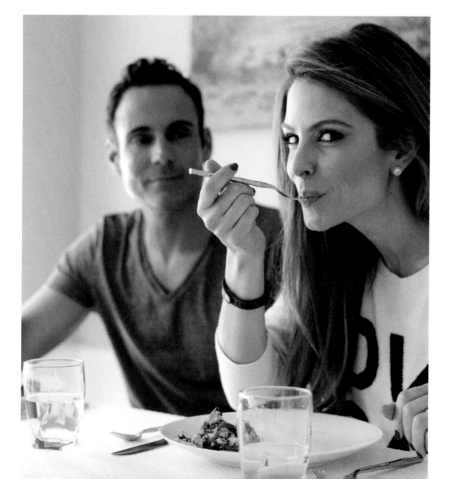

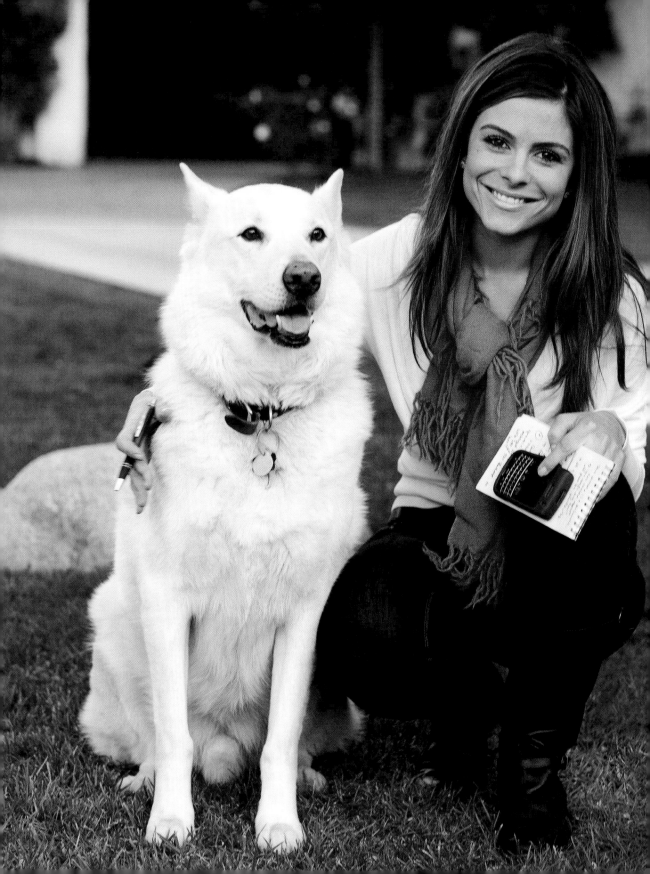

PART ONE

EveryGirl

FOUNDATION

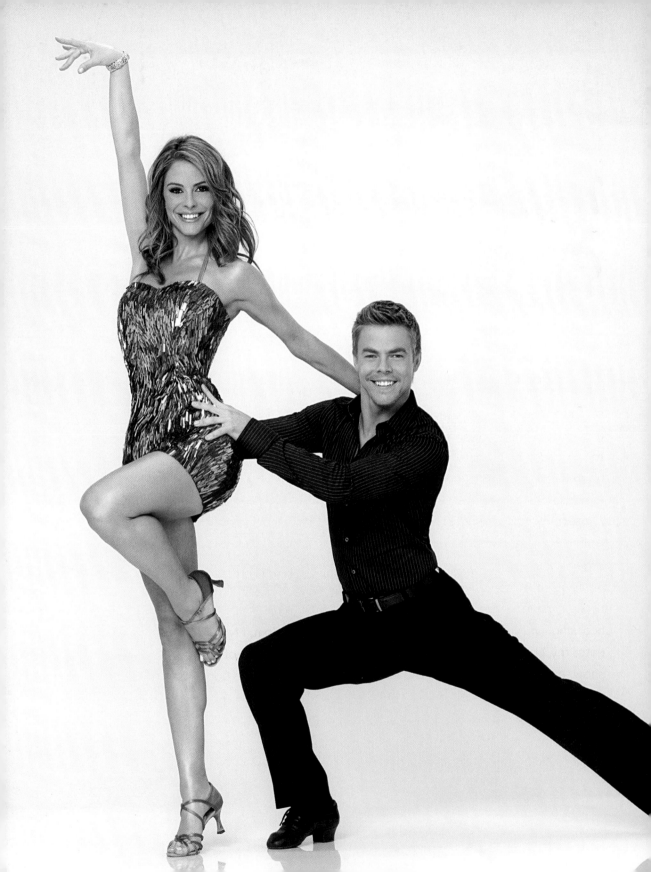

Chapter 1

My EveryGirl Journey

When ABC called and asked me to be on the hit series *Dancing with the Stars*, my first thought was, *No way*. Born with crooked legs that required metal braces and steel-reinforced shoes, I grew up as an uncoordinated kid and still have an awkward running style to this day. Nor was I much of a dancer. Growing up, I never performed in recitals the way other girls did, as my parents couldn't afford dance lessons. I didn't want to make a fool of myself in front of the whole world. And unlike some of the other *Dancing with the Stars* contestants, I had a full-time job, hosting *Extra* every day. Entertainment news is like any other news; it never stops. Would I even be able to fit in hours of rehearsing every day? At the last minute, I decided to do it. My parents; my boyfriend, Keven; and his mom were huge fans of the show, and Kev thought that the added exposure would be good for my career. It wasn't easy, emotionally or physically. I didn't learn the steps as fast as the other contestants, and I was constantly terrified that I'd mess up. I fractured both of my feet (in multiple places) and two of my ribs during our rehearsals, and I was in pain throughout. Time was tight—I hosted *Extra* every day I was dancing, and had to cram in my *Dancing with the Stars* rehearsals during the evenings. Yet for all the pain, it was one of the most rewarding experiences I've ever had; an amazing fourteen weeks learning about my body—and about my life.

Any success I had in the dancing department, I owe 100 percent to Derek Hough, my dance partner. He is the most superb dancer and a genius-level choreographer and teacher. He makes every partner look amazing. He really is that unbelievable. Derek, his parents, his sisters, and their children are like family to me, so I got a lot of emotional support, too. However, I take full credit for any success I had in terms of stamina. I owed that success to the hard lessons I'd learned in the arena of diet and fitness and the strong foundation I'd established as a result.

That foundation took years to build, and I didn't do it alone. It involved a lot of trial and error, and it certainly wasn't easy.

My Story

My parents were immigrants who came to the United States in their twenties. Before that, they lived in small villages in the mountains of Greece without electricity or running water. They could afford to eat meat only once a year, usually during holidays, so their daily meals were made up of fruits, grains, and vegetables harvested directly from their gardens.

When I was a kid, that's the way we ate pretty much all the time. My parents didn't change their diet all that much when they came to America, for two reasons. First, it was the way they liked to eat. But it was also because my dad has type 1 diabetes. We never had anything with processed sugar in the house; there were no chips, ice cream, or sugary cereals in our kitchen. I didn't even know what bagels or waffles were until late in high school. For dinner, we had a

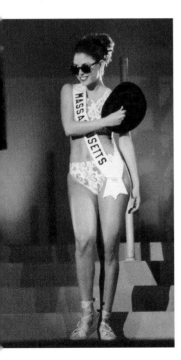

↑ Here I am at the Miss Teen USA pageant at a size 8.

THE EVERYGIRL'S GUIDE TO DIET AND FITNESS

variety of dishes made with lentils, vegetables, and beans from the garden. Our dessert? Fruit.

As a result, I was pretty thin growing up. At times my dad even worried I was *too* skinny. In the old country, being skinny was a sign that you were poor. So Dad would come home from work with the biggest chocolate bars he could find and give them to me so I could put on weight.

Then when I was thirteen, I got a job at Dunkin' Donuts. Surrounded by all that sugar, I couldn't resist indulging. (If you're not from the East Coast, you may not understand, but Dunkin' Donuts is particularly addicting. Even today, it's my first stop every time I visit Boston!) In my freshman year of high school, I was a size 3 and grew about a size every year. By senior year, I was a size 8. An important note here: Though I was gaining weight, I was definitely comfortable with my appearance. Even though I was told I was too short for a modeling career, I participated in small fashion shows, did some print work, and competed in the Miss Teen Massachusetts pageant—and yes, there was a swimsuit segment. For any of you girls who think you need to be a size 0 to be attractive, maybe you'll change your mind after I tell you that I actually *won* that pageant.

But things got worse in college. Off my parents' proverbial leash, I could keep candy and chips in my room and eat all the late-night pizza I could afford. The college cafeteria offered endless rows of all-you-can-eat fries, steak and cheese subs, sandwich melts, cake, pie, pudding, and ice cream. I had access to everything I could never have before—and I went nuts.

At my peak of overeating, I would have a bagel and cream cheese for breakfast; a large steak and cheese sandwich with lots of French fries for lunch; and ice cream, candy, and assorted junk

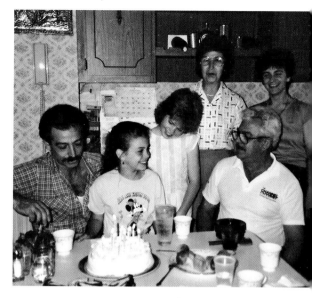

↑ This was my 11th birthday. My grandparents were visiting from Greece.

in between. I was so obsessed with brown sugar Pop-Tarts that, to this day, I won't eat them for fear that the taste will get me addicted again. At dinner, I could down a whole pizza by myself. Two hours after dinner, I would have three Eggo waffles for dessert.

Nobody could contain me.

Soon, neither could my clothes.

I grew to a size 14 and kept growing. Eating became a game to me. I started to compete with guys to see who could eat the most, and regrettably, I always won. At my heaviest, I was more than 160 pounds. Every time I came home from college, aunts, uncles, and cousins had something mean to say. They would poke fun at my size and how much weight I had gained. It hurt so much that, in defiance, I would buy a gallon of ice cream and then hide in the garage and eat it.

Looking back, I should have laughed them off, the way I hope to inspire you to do in your own battles. I don't remember thinking I looked that bad back then, and when I look at old pictures, I still don't think so. And I should have taken comfort in the fact that I was actually thriving in my life as an on-camera talent. Emerson College, my alma mater, was attended by the likes of Jay Leno, Denis Leary, Henry Winkler, and countless other showbiz heavies. They have an annual award show called the EVVY Awards for their outstanding students. I was the first freshman in the school's seventy-five-year history ever to win an EVVY for my on-camera hosting. So again, for any of you who think you need to be a size 0 to be on camera or to be beautiful, I won that award when I weighed upwards of 160 pounds and wore a size 14.

But I know how I felt: sick and lethargic. I wanted to nap all the time and struggled to get out of bed each morning. All my Emerson professors and my boyfriend, Kev, whom I had just started dating, warned me about the high level of energy and stamina I would need to work in television, especially the news. You have to be prepared

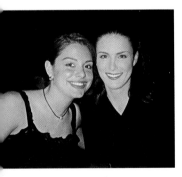

↑ In college days with my friend Jacqui Doucette. She was Miss Massachusetts USA when I was Miss Massachusetts Teen USA.

THE EVERYGIRL'S GUIDE TO DIET AND FITNESS

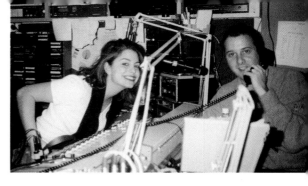

to work eighteen-hour days six to seven days a week. Their unanimous advice was if you want to make it in this business, you have to be physically fit and strong. In addition, I learned that my overeating and weight gain was putting me at greater risk for diabetes. I knew too well how the disease had affected Mom, Dad, and me. The writing was on the wall: I had to take my health and my eating habits more seriously.

↑ Not able to secure radio time at Emerson College's WERS radio station, my friend Bill Stanitsas and I started ZOH, a Greek-American radio show. Zoh, zoi, or zoe means "life" in Greek.

One Diet After Another

I tried a ton of diets—shake diets, the grapefruit diet, and the coffee diet among them—but not one of them lasted. Like the EveryGirl, I was putting in long days, trying to do it all: study, work, build a career, be a good daughter, and have a social life, too. Between my schedule and trying to make ends meet, being on a diet was just one more stress factor in an already stressful life.

An Ugly Cycle

When you're used to eating unhealthily, as I was, it's incredibly difficult, if not impossible, to do a 180-degree turnaround and follow a rigid diet plan. You're tired and you crave foods that will give you that surge of energy you desperately need. Unfortunately, they're the same foods that are loaded with junk like sugar. They do give you that jolt, but they make you crash soon after. You feel even more exhausted than before, and you reach for even more of the unhealthy food to lift you up again. It's a cyclical habit that leads to weight gain and poor health, as was clearly the case with me. And it's tough to break all at once. Is it any wonder, then, that every time I tried a new diet I'd get

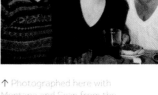

↑ Photographed here with Montana and Sean from the Real World Boston cast circa 1997.

discouraged and gradually resume my old eating habits? Trying to do a complete diet overhaul was too much to handle.

My "Diet" Discovery

Finally, in January 1999, I'd had enough. I was tired of feeling tired, getting sick all the time, and wondering why. I was tired of being out of shape, nothing fitting right, and spending way too much time trying to find clothes that would hide my flaws. Since I couldn't find a plan that worked for me, I decided to create my own. The reason the word *diet* is in quotes above is that it wasn't really an official diet. It was just me opting to set a goal and to make some dietary and lifestyle adjustments (which I'll describe in detail later). Within a year I had lost forty pounds. Little did I know that I'd stumbled on the secret to losing weight in an easy and practical way, and had found the best way to ensure I wouldn't gain it back. Things still needed a little tweaking, though.

Thinner—But Not Healthier

The newly thin me moved to California, where my career took off pretty quickly. I got a job at a place called Channel One News, a program that was beamed into high schools around the country. It was an incredible experience, and I was truly blessed to have it. However, I was working around the clock and was on the go constantly, just as Kev and my advisers had predicted. The only thing I had time for, or thought I had time for, was fast food—something that was new to me. Back in Boston, I had over indulged, but never on fast food. If you know Boston, you know there's little reason to. Boston cuisine is perhaps the most delicious in the country. There are so many local restaurants, as well as pizzerias and sub shops, with owners that have an incredible passion for their products.

Even local chains that might be considered fast food, such as Papa Gino's, Regina Pizzeria, D'Angelo's, and Boston Market, are amazing. But in L.A., I saw too few quality mom-and-pop shops and more fast-food joints than I'd ever seen in my life.

A year or so later I was hired by *Entertainment Tonight* and found myself more strapped for time than I had ever been. In my first year at *ET,* I worked fifteen-plus hours a day and forty-eight out of fifty-two weekends. And that time crunch just reinforced my fast-food habit. I'd eat it at least twice a day, often hitting the drive-through on my way to and from shoots. I bet I visited every fast-food joint in L.A.! Luckily, my weight didn't fluctuate very much. I knew enough to keep my portions small, and I was so busy working and running around that I must have burned all the calories off. Having lost the weight slowly over a year's time no doubt prevented it from piling back on, too.

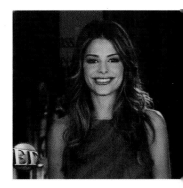

↑ In New York reporting for *Entertainment Tonight,* when I was 23.

A Final Wake-Up Call

Yet there were serious consequences to eating so much fast food, as I soon discovered. I was in and out of the hospital multiple times for exhaustion, malnutrition, and dehydration. Things got so bad that, on one occasion in France, I, literally, almost died.

I was on assignment at the Cannes Film Festival, pulling eighteen-hour days. My unhealthy diet and the exhaustion that went with it left me more susceptible to illness, and I contracted a rare intestinal infection. It was altogether painful and terrifying. I was twenty-three and found myself all alone in the corridor of a French hospital, shivering with a 105-degree fever. I didn't speak French, but it didn't take a rocket scientist to figure out that when the doctor used the words *opération chirurgicale* and *terminale,* he was talking about surgery and the possibility of death. It was the scariest experience of my life. The hospital did not want to

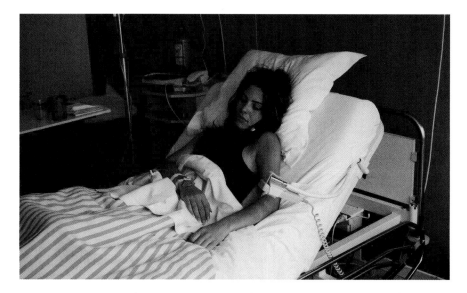

↑ My last day in the French Hospital. Tip for those who travel a lot: I got Medjet insurance after this to be flown home if seriously ill or injured while travelling.

release me, but I knew I had to return home. Keven didn't have a passport to come get me, but he spoke enough French to persuade hospital officials to release me once the fever got down to 102. He urged me to find the strength to get on a plane; I basically crawled onto the flight.

Rachel to the Rescue

When I finally got home and told my best friend, Rachel Zalis, what had happened, she was the one who made the connection between my unhealthy eating habits and how they were affecting my health. Rachel, then the West Coast editor at *Glamour* magazine and today a top style expert, knew some of the world's leading diet and health practitioners. More important, she had grown up in a family of doctors. Rachel has never eaten fast food in her life, and she advised me to stop eating it, too. I cut out that junk food entirely for a few years and never got sick as a result—not even a cold. Today, I'll have fast food on occasion for fun, but it is not and never again will be a staple of my diet.

The Most Important Lesson

It was through that life-or-death experience in France that I realized the whole quest to have an amazing body or to be skinny needed to be seriously reevaluated. The end goal should not be "having a better body." What the hell does that matter if you're dead or immobile? It's about living a healthy life—with the wonderful by-product being that "better body." Just because you are thinner, does not mean you are healthier.

I made it my mission to figure out the very best ways to control my weight and be healthy at the same time. My job as a reporter and host for such outlets as the *Today* show, *Access Hollywood*, NBC *Nightly News*, and now *Extra* gave me the opportunity to interview the world's leading diet, fitness, and health experts. By combining their advice with the healthy eating lessons I had learned as a child, I found my way to a fit and healthy body.

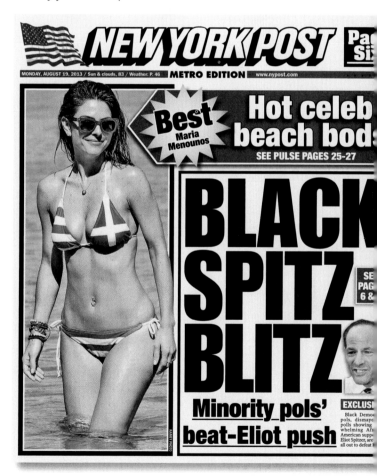

Putting It to a Vote

In a poll just last year, the online readers of the E! channel were asked who had the ultimate bikini body—and they picked me. I was stunned; I swear I never thought I'd be praised for my body—ever. The praise was nice, but even better, the honor affirmed my belief that my EveryGirl approach is the

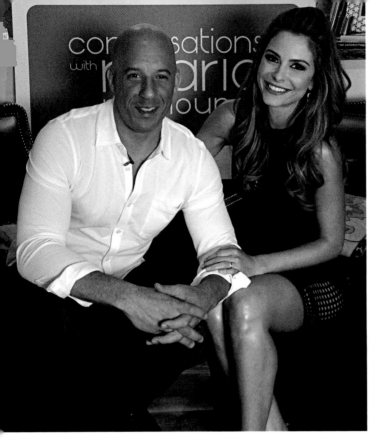

↑ On set of my online talk show *Conversations with Maria Menounos* with my dear friend Vin Diesel.

right approach, even in a town where people are working out daily with the best trainers and adhering to the strictest of diets.

In truth, I'm not as fit, toned, and muscular as many of the stars out here; given that I was once forty pounds heavier, we know that I wasn't born with a great metabolism. But when it comes to working at my job(s) and accomplishing my daily tasks, I have a stamina that's equal to, if not greater than, the best of them. And, knock on wood, I'm healthy and strong. Yet I don't work out two hours a day. I don't even work out every day or rely on a weekly trainer. Between hosting *Extra* and *Conversations with Maria Menounos;* serving as CEO of the largest online broadcast network, AfterBuzzTV.com; and writing books, not to mention other side jobs and projects, I'm way too busy. I also have my parents, my boyfriend, my dogs, my staff, and my loved ones who rely on me.

On top of all that, I'm human, and I like to let loose. I don't follow many of the traditional "rules" that some diet gurus swear by. I drink beer and love ordering appetizers at places like Chili's and TGI Fridays. I love watching TV and movies and socializing with friends. By coming up with a customizable plan that lets me take all these factors into consideration, I'm not at the mercy of someone else's definition of the "right" way to be healthy. I'm in a position to make smart choices that work for me. And so can you.

THE EVERYGIRL'S GUIDE TO DIET AND FITNESS

No Time? No Money? No Problem!

Without time or money, I succeeded in losing weight. Later, with education and experience but no more time or money, I got healthy. I'm not telling you this to brag—I'm telling you this to inspire. Perhaps you don't think you have as many jobs as I do, but I'd argue, *Yes, you do!* And if you're a mother, you have way more on your plate than I do. (If that weren't true, I'd be a mother myself by now!) If you're a single working girl, you're under a lot of pressure, too. And whether you're a single working girl or a mom or anything in between, society puts so much pressure on us to be everything to everyone and, of course, to look our best.

I know that, like me, nearly all of you are in the same position and have to live up to all that and cram so many tasks into your days to make it all work. The blessings of technology can also be a curse—everything moves so fast today! That's why I think the Every-Girl way is the best way, even if you happen to have the resources to hire a trainer and a personal chef. Sure, these days I'm in a better position financially, but I'm also extremely frugal. (I'm so bad that my dad, who is very frugal in his own right, teases me about it.) The truth is, a career in Hollywood has a short shelf life, so I have to save as much as I can (the way the economy has been, we *all* have to be more careful with the money we have). For all of those reasons, when it comes to diet and fitness, I still act as though I don't have very much money at all!

My Foundation: My Family

Whether it's the family you are born with or the one you create along the way, a good family is the basis of good health. My family is no exception. They are such a huge part of my foundation, inspiration, and strength. Each of them in one way or another has influenced

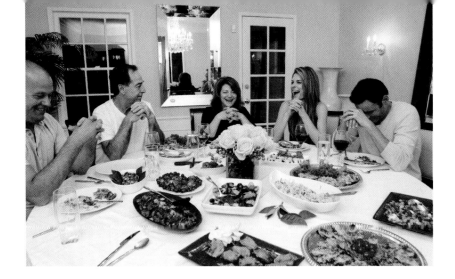

my diet and fitness education and journey. And by introducing them to you, I hope that they'll be a positive influence for you, too.

Costas the Greek!

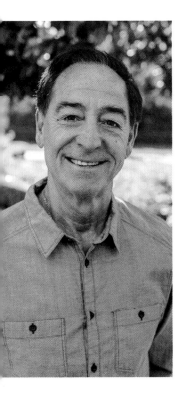

I adore my father like any child should any good father, but that's not the main reason you'll find me continually referencing him in the book. The truth is that my father, Costas, encapsulates the very essence of this book—that even with no time and no money, long-term fitness and health is possible.

As I said, both Mom and Dad were immigrants who raised me on a Greek Mediterranean diet that focused mainly on fresh fruits and vegetables grown from our garden. Mediterranean diets are trendy now, and there are many studies that show they can help you lose weight, prevent heart disease, improve your memory, and more. (In fact, one study found that people eating Mediterranean-style food lost between four and nine pounds more on average than people who tried a weight-loss diet.) In addition, some of the longest-living people hail from cultures that subsist on Mediterranean diets. But my parents didn't know that then. More than anything, Mom and Dad just had a common-sense approach to life and problems. Like most immigrants, they knew how to adapt quickly—which came in handy when dealing with my dad's type 1 diabetes. Even though they worked as unskilled laborers, didn't speak English, and certainly didn't get the best health care early on, they both learned that processed sugars were bad and that high-carbohydrate foods like bread, potatoes, pasta, and rice act like sugar in the body. Hearing that was all it took for Dad to summon his willpower and resist all of those foods. For years, he consumed mainly fresh fruit, vegetables, whole grains, fish, and (very little) lean meat. Despite forty-five-plus years with type 1 diabetes, Dad shows little to none of the disease's common complications, such as loss of vision or nerve damage, or the circulation problems that sometimes lead to limb amputation. One of my dad's doctors in Boston was so impressed by his condition that he sent my father's lab reports to his colleagues at MIT. When they read them, they immediately requested

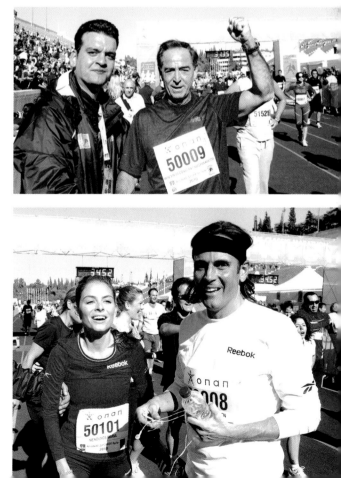

↓ With my dad at the Greek Marathon 5K. Check out his time, 31:35, and mine, 34:52— and I look beat! He beat us all!

Dad come in for a study. Last year, when we ran a road race together in Greece, *he* beat *me*!

That should tell you that Dad is very fit and toned, but he doesn't rely on weight lifting or jogging. Instead, he's in constant movement. A lot of his day is spent being active, doing things like yard work and chores, and when he moves, he *moves*. He always opts for walking rather than driving or taking stairs over elevators. He doesn't stroll to and from the tool shed; he walks at a brisk pace. During the winter, when it's too cold back east to work in the yard, he might, while watching the Boston Bruins games, play around with the resistance bands and light dumbbells that Kev got him. But the main thing is he's consciously and constantly moving in everything he does. Sometimes while working, he'll listen to Greek music on his iPod and sing and dance out loud as he does. And if you think he sounds boring and not someone an EveryGirl can relate to, at parties he dances all night and loves to drink red wine and tequila. He even distills his own red wine at our house in Connecticut. Put simply, he found a "plan" that worked for him, not a rigid diet or exercise program.

His eating and fitness regimens keep him toned and trim but also young. At almost seventy, an age when many people are popping all kinds of pills and moving slowly, Costas has the most incredible quality of life. All the twenty-something employees at our AfterBuzz TV studios marvel at how much more energy he has than they do. His retirement is what it's supposed to be: a time to have fun and do all the things he couldn't afford to do when he was younger.

If we all mirrored my dad's behavior, in many ways we may not need this diet and fitness book or any other one. We probably wouldn't even need as many doctors. But like all of us, he's not perfect with his health, either. Sometimes he gets carried away with work and forgets to check his blood sugar, which can run dangerously low, to the point he risks falling into a coma or having a heart attack. Yet, he prioritizes his health every day. Although I don't have his willpower, his is an excellent example to aspire to.

Litsa the Great

As they say, behind every great man stands a great woman. In the case of my mother, Litsa, they couldn't be more right. Mom was not only the daughter of a Greek chef but also a professional cook for an elementary and middle school cafeteria. Responsible for pushing out some two thousand meals a day, my mom's efforts helped her school's breakfast and lunch program ascend from the state's lowest ranked school to the state's highest. Mom specialized in Greek Mediterranean cuisine, which, as I said, is one of the healthiest in the world. At home, she cooked meals with produce from our garden and, to help Dad with his diabetes, became creative in the kitchen, devising some of the healthiest and most sumptuous meals you can imagine. Her incredible talents in the kitchen have guaranteed that our family eats healthily without *ever* feeling as though we are sacrificing on taste. As Keven says, only Litsa can make vegetables taste so amazing. But now you will be able to as well. Her recipes are included later in the book! Mom definitely doesn't have my dad's willpower when it comes to food, though. She loves to indulge and struggles to avoid overdoing it with portion sizes and sweets. But to compensate, she is every bit as active as my dad is, maybe even more so. She is constantly running errands, cooking, cleaning, and fixing things alongside my father.

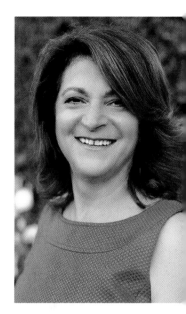

Keven the BF

As some of you know, Keven and I have been together fifteen years. Just like my mom has been in my dad's corner all these years, Kev has been in mine. When I was nineteen and trying to produce movies, it was Kev who told me that I was on the wrong side of the camera and that I'd be a huge and famous success in Hollywood if I ever got in front of it. When I began working out for the Miss Massachusetts pageant, Kev helped me train and stretch, and he massaged my muscles every night when I was done. He still gives the best massages, which come in handy after I've been standing in heels for fourteen hours! With Kev, I joke that I live with my ice-skating coach, because he pushes me that hard. But the truth is, he's my biggest champion. He believes in me like no one else and is determined to see me succeed and to be healthy and happy.

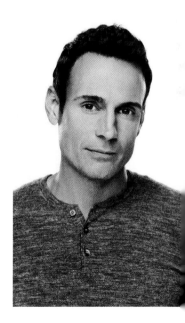

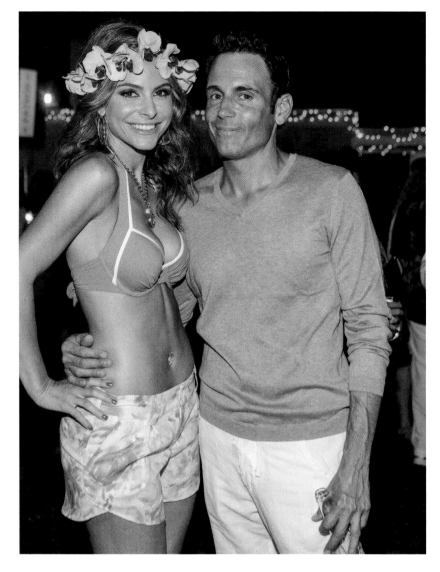

Kev worked many summers as a carnival worker as a means to travel to Los Angeles each winter to write for television. (He helped me write my first book, and he helped me write this one.) The TV writing part was easy for him, including being a head writer for MTV. Being a "carny," not so much. It meant working fourteen- to twenty-hour days pretty much seven days a week. The working conditions were also some of the most brutal and unhealthy. I know because I worked alongside him one season. Yet despite all that, Kev, like my parents, managed to discover unique ways to remain healthy and fit. If I'm EveryGirl, Kev is EveryGuy. Though he works in Hollywood and is very successful, most of the time he prefers to drive a secondhand truck, wear work boots and Levi's, and do most of our house repairs and renovations himself. He works fifteen hours a day on average and

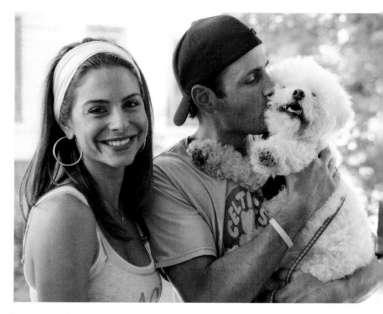

would work seven days a week if I didn't stop him. It isn't easy to fit workouts in, but he figured out how. Three mornings a week he spends less than thirty minutes using resistance bands, dumbbells, and other home equipment. He has *never* hired a trainer, yet he's gotten great results in part because he's constantly seeking out new and better exercises, routines, and methods. He has a ton of energy. While all the younger people are huffing and puffing with their hands on their knees during hoop games at our house, Kev is running circles around them, talking trash, and cracking jokes. We both love to veg out together and binge-watch our favorite TV shows, but we also play basketball, hike, and walk the dogs together, too, all of which helps us stay in shape and remain close as a couple.

Unlike my dad's diet, Kev's could use some work. He either forgets to eat or, when he does, eats on the run. He loves soda and candy, too, but knows he needs to work on that.

My parents and Kev are great examples of people who do their best to make fitness work without much time or money.

Nobody's Perfect

Dad runs his sugar levels low, Mom overindulges with food, and Kev's diet is erratic. My family isn't perfect, but I think that's what makes them aspirational. (Despite what you see of me on TV or in magazines, I also have my unhealthy ways that I still need to work on—believe me.) We've just had more success in diet and fitness than failure in our lives, but like you, we remain works in progress. If you don't have a lot of time or money to get in shape, or you think you have perpetual bad habits you struggle to break like we do, I got you.

My Extended Family

While my immediate family profoundly inspired so many elements of this book, my extended family did as well. Two of them specifically have graciously and tirelessly shared their philosophies, techniques, success, and knowledge. They helped contribute so much to this book and, more than anything, to my life. I believe you will prosper as much from their expertise as I do.

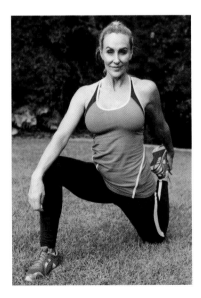

ANDREA ORBECK is a celebrity trainer, fitness expert, former Olympian, and pregnancy fitness specialist who's sculpted some of the world's most beautiful bodies from Heidi Klum, Karolina Kurkova, and other supermodels to Seal and Usher. Andrea is the creator and star of the bestselling DVDs *Supermodel Sculpt* and *Pregnancy Sculpt* and has been featured in *Elle, Self, Shape, Glamour, Fitness, Us Weekly, Allure,* and *OK!* magazines, among others; and she recently spoke at the 2013 TED Conferences. See more at *andreaorbeck.com*.

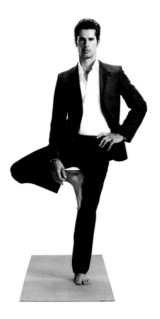

CAMERON ALBORZIAN is one of the leading figures in yoga and Ayurvedic therapy who offers natural medicines and treatments to help people live a healthier and happier life. Yogi Cameron trained at the Integral Yoga Institute in New York City, and in India at Arsha Yoga, where he studied Ayurveda for five years. He's the author of *The One Plan* and *The Guru in You* and the host of *A Model Guru* on Veria Living TV. His celeb clients include Ellen DeGeneres, and he's appeared on *The Ellen DeGeneres Show, Extra,* and the *Today* show and in *Glamour, Elle, GQ, Allure,* and *Vogue*. See more at *yogicameron.com*.

EveryGirl's Guide to Diet and Fitness

In this book, I'm going to show how you, the EveryGirl, can find your best and healthiest body and get where you want to be—without having to give up the things you truly love. I'll outline the major principles I have for eating, exercise, and overall health, and I'm going to give you recipes, workouts, and tools that you can use. But there are three important points I want to make first.

➔ I'm not a certified trainer, dietitian, or nutritionist, and I have no medical training whatsoever. I believe that, for the purposes of this book, I am something better: an EveryGirl who grew up in a blue-collar environment and once put on forty pounds too many. Then, with limited resources, I took the weight off and kept it off *before* I got to Hollywood. And when

I got to Hollywood, I ran myself down and was hospitalized and compromised my health. From there I made adjustments and picked the brains of every expert I could find while engaging in further health, diet, and fitness trials and tribulations. I'm not an expert—I'm just someone who's been through it and who wants to share her experience so that maybe you will achieve success while avoiding the mistakes I made along the way.

➜ I define *diet* as a loose plan for healthy yet realistic eating habits every day for the rest of your life. I hate the word *diet* when it's used to denote a temporary plan designed for weight loss, as in, "I'm going on a diet." When used this way, it just puts more pressure on you and in most cases serves as a short-term solution. My goal isn't to give you a one-size-fits-all prescription that involves eating kiwi at 9:30 a.m. and then a four-ounce piece of salmon for dinner with three asparagus spears, or some specific rule-book on how it *must* be done. What I want to do is give you the principles and strategies that can work in your life—that you can adjust depending on your own needs and situations. I'll give some structure for those who crave it, and I'll give flexibility for those who don't. But what I most want to give you is the power to make gradual changes that you can stick to—not just for today, tomorrow, and until your motivation runs out, but for the rest of your long and healthy life.

➜ Trainers, dietitians, and doctors all have different beliefs when it comes to diet and fitness. Sometimes they overlap, and sometimes they contradict each other. Many of them think that their way is the only way to go. While it's true that there are certain undeniable facts on diet and fitness, there is much that *is* speculative. Each person's body and mind respond differently to different techniques and foods. What helps one person lose weight or tone up may not help someone else quite as much. Similarly, there will be some suggestions and observations in this book that you'll agree with or be motivated to try, and there'll be some that you won't. That's okay. I'm constantly switching workouts around, learning new things, and taking different approaches. The idea is to be open-minded and to discover habits and a lifestyle that work for you.

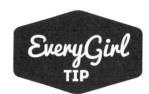

PROOF ON DIETING

UCLA researchers looked at thirty-one diet studies, and what they found was shocking: Dieting was actually the number one predictor of future weight gain!

If diets don't work, then is lasting weight loss hopeless? No! I'm proof of that. What does work, experts say, is eating healthily most of the time. That means eating a balanced diet composed primarily of foods that come from the ground.

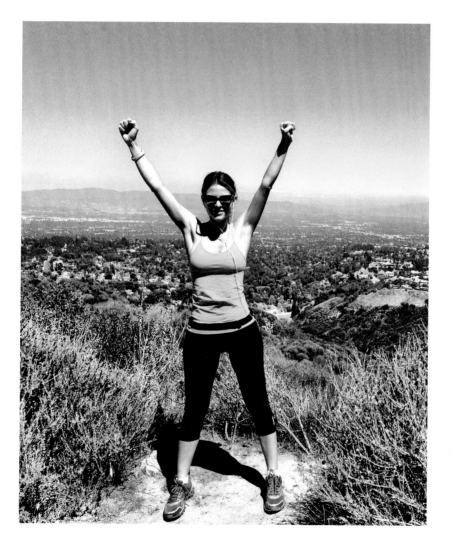

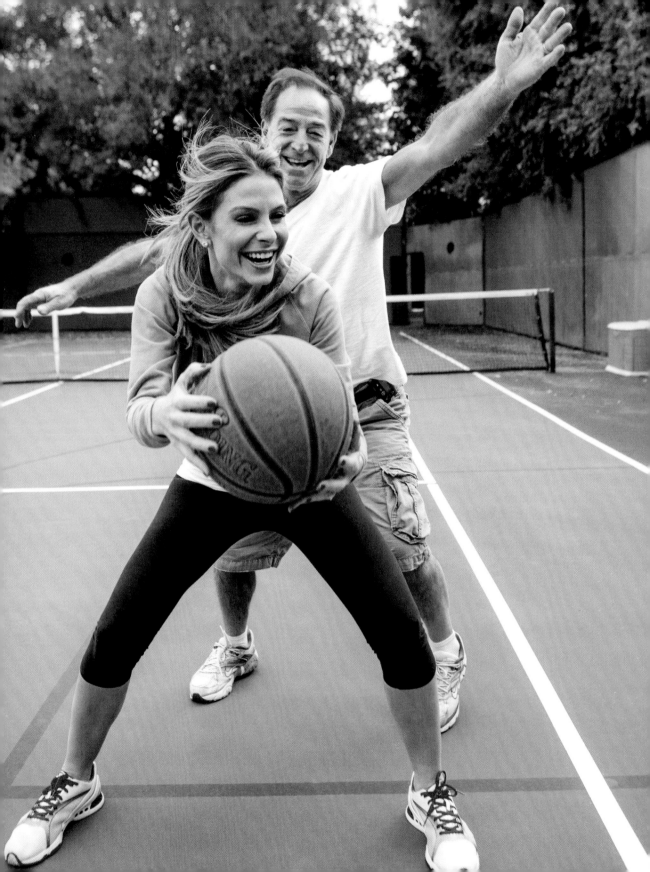

Chapter 2

The Fifty-Year Plan

What started as a running joke between Kev and me is actually now a useful tool. When I'd leave dishes in the sink, as I often did, Kev would say, "You gotta get on the fifty-year plan." And when Kev would leave cabinet doors and drawers open, as he often did, I'd say the same thing back. The translation was that we had to work on those issues, and other bigger ones, if in fact we wanted to be together for the next fifty years—which, of course, we do. For a relationship to be sustainable, you have to focus on the little everyday things that will help not just now but also in the long run.

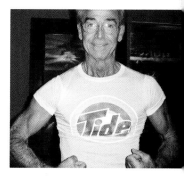

↑ This is without traditional workouts. This is pure, clean eating and physical labor.

The same fifty-year philosophy should be applied to fitness and health. If we want to be healthy and maintain a high quality of life over the next fifty years, what are the things we can do today to make that happen?

The fifty-year plan doesn't simply mean living another fifty years. Plenty of people do that, and with catastrophic outcomes. They spend those later years sick, tired, or unhappy. When I say get on the fifty-year plan, I mean take steps now to improve the *quality* of the life you'll have in the present and in the future. The fifty-year plan not only makes it much more likely that you'll live to be ninety-plus but that you'll do it while still being active and effective in daily life. One of the many reasons that my father embodies the essential message of this book is that he's on the fifty-year plan.

My dad's goal is to be just as active in his nineties as he is now, and if we can keep his blood sugar levels from dropping, God willing, he's on track to do so. Don't be cynical and believe it's not possible to have quality of life in old age or that it's all in your genes. Some people say that it's in my dad's genes to thrive health-wise. But that's a cynical outlook, and it upsets him so much because it discredits all the hard work and smart choices he's made to be healthy.

When it comes to deciding how to eat or how physically active to be, it's important to think in the back of your head what it will all mean fifty years from now. But that's not all it's about. The fifty-year plan applies to curbing certain exercises and activities that stress your body and leave you susceptible to injury. For example, if you like running long distances but are experiencing worse and worse back and knee pains, what will that mean fifty years from now if you continue? More than likely you won't be able to walk, or you'll need hip and knee replacements. It may be time to switch to something that has less impact on your joints, like swimming or the elliptical machine.

I don't see the fifty-year plan as a luxury or just another option. It's easy to think that we're never going to get old or that pills and modern medicine will take care of everything. Or maybe you think you won't care—you'll be happy being wheeled around when you're seventy. Believe me, that's not the case. Time really does fly, and with people living longer, you don't want to spend the last twenty or thirty years of your life sick or immobile. And at the same time we're living longer in an economy that may seem like it's stabilizing, but really doesn't offer the brightest of futures. We make fewer

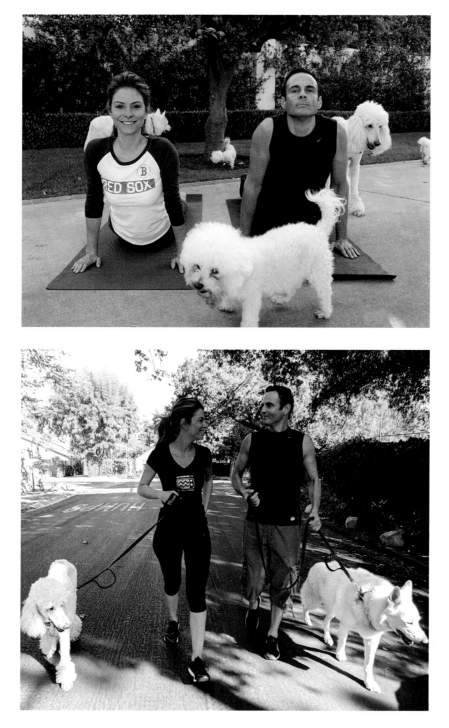

← Sometimes I force Kev to do some yoga with me... The dogs like to get in the way.

↙ We love walking our dogs. It's a great time to talk and a good way to keep accumulating steps.

products in America today than we used to and outsource much of our labor to other countries. I know, you're asking, "How is that relevant to diet and fitness, Maria?" Well, think about it: How can a weak economy support people retiring at age fifty-five or sixty-two, who may need expensive health care and live another twenty-five to thirty-five years? I believe the EveryGirl will have to be strong, mobile, independent, and pulling her own weight in her sixties and beyond.

Before you think I'm painting a picture of doom and gloom, the amazing news is that most people *can* be like my dad. In fact, I know plenty of people in their sixties, seventies, and even older who are still working or contributing in some way. The people who make it a point to stay relevant are the happiest people of all. Many of us just have a misconception about work—the same misconception about eating right and exercising, I suspect. For the sake of the next fifty years of your life and many years beyond, I hope we can change that.

Jack LaLanne: The Fifty-Plus-Year Plan

Long before my friends Jillian Michaels and Harley Pasternak came on the scene, there was a man by the name of Jack LaLanne. Known as the "Godfather of Fitness," Jack was the world's first famous trainer and fitness guru. Jumping jacks were named after him, and he invented several pieces of strength equipment that are still in use today. In 1936, at the age of twenty-one, he opened what were probably the nation's first modern health spas. Jack also had a TV fitness show that ran nationally from the 1950s to the 1980s. Certainly, Jack was on his own version of the fifty-year plan! If all that's not enough to make Jack relevant to the messages in this book, he was also the first person to encourage women not only to join his gym but also to lift weights and to be strong—even though he was thoroughly criticized for it at the time.

I didn't know about any of this until I met Jack, back when I worked for *Entertainment Tonight*. He was ninety and still had such a passion for health above anything else and for helping people achieve it. His exuberant, positive energy and the way he was so present, commanding, and active at ninety, as if he were fifty, had me in awe and left a permanent impression on me.

Jack believed that our habits make us fat, not other factors like our father's bad genes. According to Jack, if we are overweight, it is because we eat garbage or are inactive, plain and simple. Nobody forces that food down our throats. We have to take responsibility for ourselves. Jack used himself as an example. He said that as a boy, he was addicted to sugar and that he suffered headaches and acted out violently. When he cleaned up his diet, his health improved. And when processed foods came onto the market, he shunned them, saying, "If man made it, I don't eat it." He blamed processed foods for many of our health problems and believed that sugar, salt, artificial food additives, preservatives, and flavorings as well as drugs contribute to umpteen physical and mental illnesses. He believed that people then turn to things like drugs and alcohol to cope.

Similarly, in Jack's opinion, many of our aches and illnesses like constipation, insomnia, fatigue, anxiety, high blood pressure, and depression are just symptoms of the real problem: lack of physical activity.

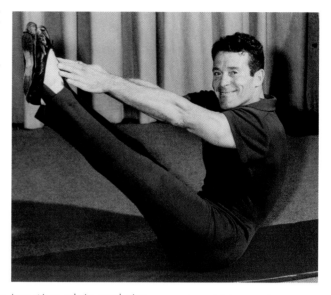

↑ Jack LaLanne in his prime

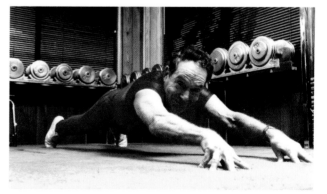

↓ Jack LaLanne living the fifty-year plan.

Jack wanted to inspire and teach everyone to be more active, not just with formal exercise, but in daily life, too. Overall, he wasn't as much about helping people build muscle and lose weight as he was about helping people to get healthy and just helping people in general.

He wasn't into long, complicated exercise routines. Jack said you could get fit in as little as twenty minutes, three times a week. His workouts involved simple exercises using things you have around the house, such as chairs and rugs. Fifty years ago, he used an elastic cord called the Glamour Stretcher, the precursor to resistance bands. He thought warmups were a waste of time (why not spend those fifteen minutes actually exercising?) and advocated switching up your routine frequently. And he didn't believe in taking breaks during exercise, either. He just kept moving. In fact, Jack worked out the day before he died at the age of ninety-six. He was sick for a week but refused to see a doctor. If he had, maybe he'd still be here.

As I think about my father pushing seventy and the diet and fitness principles we both subscribe to, I see how amazingly similar they are to Jack LaLanne's. Jack and Costas even had the same diet habits. Just like Dad, Jack first cut back on meat and then gave it up entirely, sticking to fresh fish, fruits, vegetables, whole grains, legumes, and nuts.

My dad, a man who's had type 1 diabetes for forty-five years, is proud of his fitness level, saying in his thick Greek accent, "I am . . . like bull!" And I lost forty pounds and kept it off doing pretty much what Jack advocated all those years ago. My father, my mother, Kev, and I all live by similar principles, so we know that they work. But Jack *proved* they really work. In addition to getting to know great fitness teachers like Harley Pasternak, Jillian Michaels, and Andrea Orbeck, I count meeting Jack and learning from him as one of my many blessings.

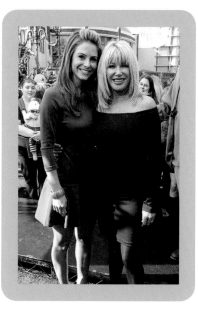

Q **What is your best advice for someone struggling to lose weight?**

Stop dieting! This futile, endless merry-go-round so many women find themselves on is frustrating, debilitating, and, frankly, no fun. Instead, eat real food: If you can pick it, pluck it, milk it, or shoot it, you can eat it.

Q **What is your philosophy on health?**

I choose health. It's a daily commitment. In order to benefit, it has to matter to you, or you will never do what is required to stay healthy. Poor health is miserable and it takes the joy out of life.

Q **What's one food people should consider removing from their diet and one they should consider adding?**

Never drink diet soda! And add coconut oil.

Q **What is one thing in your diet you realized you should change, and how did the change help/affect you?**

I took the EnteroLab stool test (I know, gross). But it is the greatest way to determine your food allergies and intolerances. I found out I was horribly allergic to egg whites and egg yolks. It actually said, "Avoid forever." I gave up eggs and I lost ten pounds in two weeks, and my bloating went away. My energy also improved. With the environmental assault of modern life, all of us are very affected by food allergies and chemical sensitivities. Eliminating that which your body perceives as "poison" to you improves your quality of life.

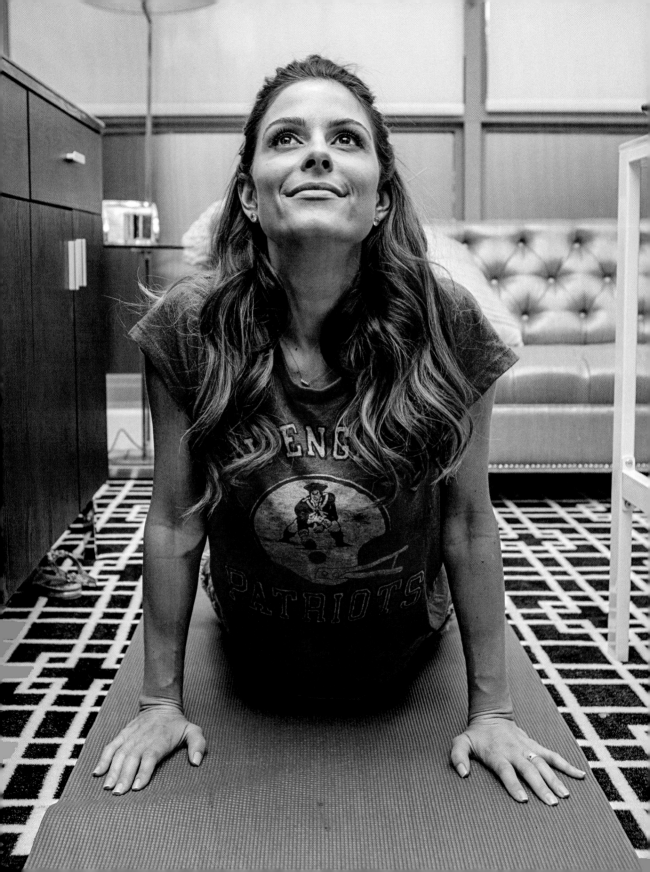

Chapter 3

A House Can't Be Built on Sand... Neither Can a Body!

I began my first book and *New York Times* bestseller, *The EveryGirl's Guide to Life,* by explaining the importance of having a strong foundation in your life. That's what will help you accomplish tasks and achieve goals, including those related to a healthy body. You can build the most amazing and beautiful house, but if the foundation of that structure, the base upon which the house rests, is made of sand instead of cement, it will surely collapse. The same can be said for your body. Chances are that if, up to now, you've gained weight and can't lose it, or are unhealthy or unhappy with your body, your foundation isn't strong.

I don't know of any task or goal more difficult than the ones involved in improving your health. There are certainly none more worthy. But while changing the way you eat and exercise might get you the metaphorical "home" of your dreams in the form of an ideal

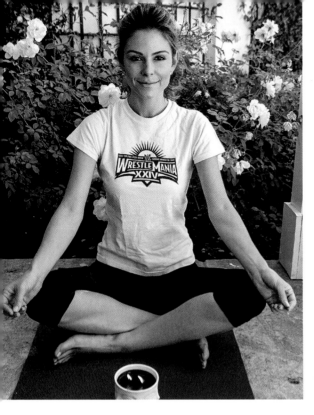

body (whatever that means to you), if you have a weak foundation, the change won't be sustainable. The foundation of that new body will be made of sand, and you'll "collapse" back into your old habits. What I want is for you to strengthen your foundation so that the changes you make and the body you get as a result of those changes will be built to last.

There are two cornerstones of your foundation that you should inspect and, if necessary, bulk up before you even *think* about changing the way you eat or exercise: the emotional and the physical aspects of your life.

Emotionally, you need to distance yourself as best you can from negative feelings such as guilt, resentment, and anger as well as surround yourself with healthy people who are positive and rooting for your success. Physically, you need your surroundings and environments to be as uncluttered and organized as possible. I can assure you that if you take time to get these areas in order at the start, the eating and exercise changes will be a whole lot easier. The benefit: a healthy body and happy soul.

So before I get into the details of how EveryGirl should eat and exercise, I want to explain the steps to take and the things to think about to help get your emotional and physical foundations in order.

The Importance of Balance

How many times have you heard the phrase "You need to have a balanced diet." Surely, *balance* doesn't apply just to diet; it applies to everything in life. Just as your diet doesn't have to be made up of only fruits and vegetables, working out doesn't have to be an hour and a half a day, seven days a week. Your career doesn't have to consume every waking hour. You don't have to give every minute of your free time to others. Your house doesn't have to be immaculate. You don't have to be pencil thin. You get the picture. With all of those issues and pretty much every other one in life, you just need balance. Balance is an essential component of a healthy and strong foundation. Let's keep that in mind as we build ours.

EMOTIONAL FOUNDATION

Recently, I hosted a girls' weekend with two of my cousins. Both were like sisters to me growing up. Both have great jobs and are married with children. Besides my missing them terribly, I invited them out for a visit because all three of us had endured some form of health crisis. For me, it was a flare-up of a stress rash. So I set us up with a bunch of consultations and treatments. First on my list: Yogi Cameron, an Ayurvedic healer. Years before, Cameron had helped me cure a rash that covered my body, after I had tried steroid creams and steroid pills—with worsening results. I also asked another holistic healer, Vicky Vlachonis (who is Greek, coincidentally), to help us out as well.

My cousins had neck, back, and other skin issues, so I lined up treatments with Dr. Michael Sheps, who did laser therapy on my fractured feet during *Dancing with the Stars*. Laser provides deep heat to relieve pain in aching joints. For other joint ailments, we also did cryo-freeze treatments with my friends Dr. Jonas and Emilia

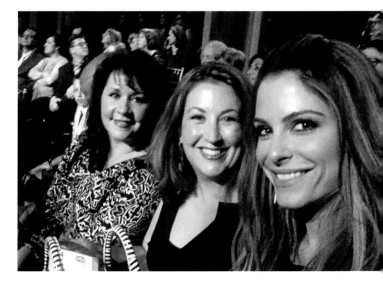

↓ With my cousins Nikki and Elaine at *Dancing with the Stars.*

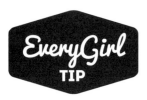

EveryGirl TIP

LASER THERAPY

Laser therapy is a non-invasive and virtually painless procedure used worldwide to treat acute and chronic pain and inflammation. Lasers penetrate deep into injured tissue and stimulate the reproduction of healthy and uninjured cells that relieve pain and accelerate rehabilitation. It is used as a safe alternative to cortisone and other pain medications, which can have severe side effects. For more information about Dr. Sheps and laser therapy, please visit *allbackandjointcare.com*.

Kuehne. Cryo got me through *Dancing with the Stars* and is so effective that many people involved in the show use it to this day, as do many professional athletes all over the world. My dad uses it to cure stiffness or pain in his back and knees. You basically step into a freezing chamber for a couple of minutes. It's not expensive considering the results, which are amazing.

We hit up my friend Nurse Jamie in Santa Monica for laser and spa treatments. We also went out and had a good time at the Soho House in West Hollywood for dinner, where we hung with Sofia Vergara—who wanted to know all about our girls' health retreat weekend! Throughout the weekend, we reminisced, vented, shared, laughed, and cried to one other. It was wonderful to spend that time with them, but also from a broader perspective, *so* much more was revealed to me and to them about what we as women internalize, struggle with, and endure and how much of that compromises our health.

I had invited my cousins out because I knew they were hurting and because I wanted to help, but, in so doing, they were the ones who helped me—as is so often the case when any of us help others. Here's what we found out.

EveryGirl Is Guilty

I mean EveryGirl *feels* guilty—or most of us do, anyhow—about a number of different issues. My cousins and I, for example, feel that we are never doing enough for our partners, our children, our parents, our in-laws, our friends, our bosses, our co-workers, etc.—everyone! We women, in general, put way more pressure on ourselves to be perfect and to please others than guys do. And society puts more pressure on us in return, too. In different areas where guys get a pass, so much more is expected of us. And this pressure takes a vicious toll. We eat poorly, don't take time for

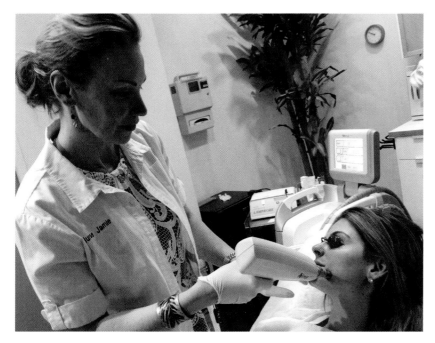

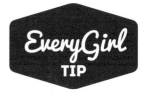

← This laser nurse Jamie is using on me is called Clearlift Q-Switch Pixel. The non-ablative laser creates thousands of microscopic perforations in the surface of the skin. The area around each of these tiny perforations is intact and allows the skin to heal rapidly by producing new collagen and leaving the skin smooth as glass.

EveryGirl TIP

CRYOTHERAPY

Whole body cryotherapy is the process of exposing the entire body to ultra-low temperatures (approximately -240°F) for two minutes. Used in Japan in 1978 to treat rheumatoid arthritis, WBC has been certified by European studies as a powerful treatment for inflammatory disorders and injuries and a boost to the body's metabolic rate, which accelerates weight loss outcomes. Professional athletes have discovered WBC to be a powerful treatment to decrease recovery time, too. As I write this book, cryotherapy is only available in Los Angeles, but I'm positive that word will spread about how effective it is and centers will start popping up all over the country.

ourselves to exercise and rejuvenate, and just let our health slide. Oftentimes, deep down, I swear women don't feel they even deserve to be happy.

Is it any wonder that it takes a major illness or a loved one's insistence to force us to slow down and think of ourselves? There's an argument to be made that, in some cases, we actually get sick, subconsciously, just to get a break. I either have to be covered in a rash and feel like my body is engulfed in flames or have Kev say, "You need to stop and get to bed!" before I put myself first. And I know it's not just me. My cousins and many of my girlfriends are the same way.

The only reason we even allowed ourselves to take that weekend was because we all had illnesses. It's sad that three hard-working women are so practical-minded and guilt-ridden that we don't think we should be able to get away and do something just for fun! It's something that we, and maybe you, too, need to work on. If you do have feelings of guilt, know that it's

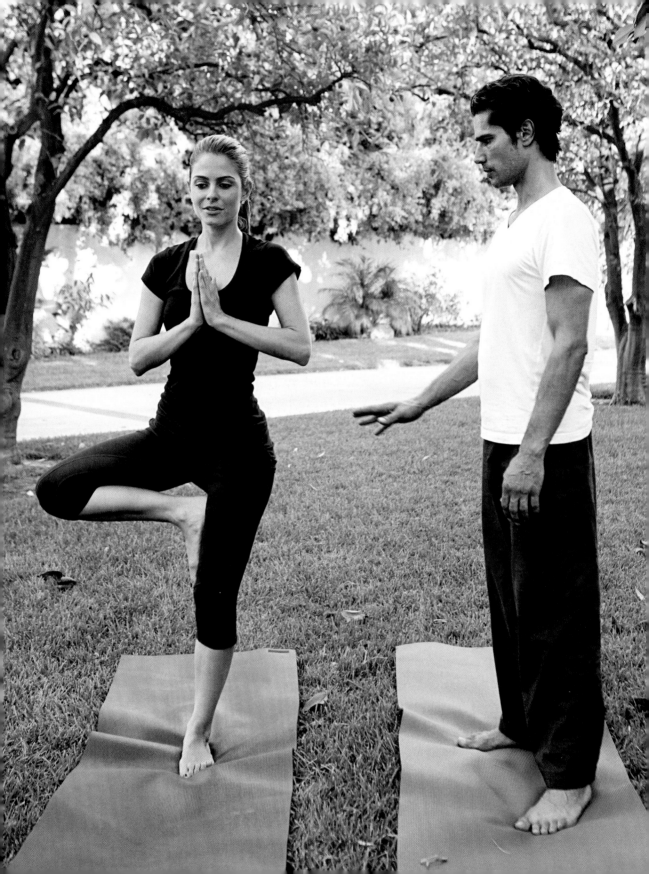

most likely contributing heavily to your being out of shape or in poor health. But also recognize that you don't need to feel guilty if you take time for and think of yourself. You're not good to anyone if you get run down.

EveryGirl Is Afraid

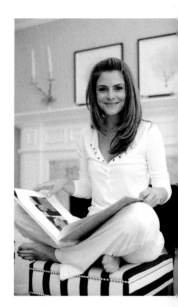

I'm afraid if I don't work hard enough, I may lose my house and not be able to support my parents. I also used to live in daily fear that my dad would die from his diabetes. My cousins had similar worries. All of us have fears of failure or even fears beyond those fears. Some of us are even afraid to be happy, as if in so doing we are going to jinx ourselves and something bad will happen as a result. This all puts more crippling pressure on us and surely has the same debilitating effects that guilt does.

EveryGirl Bottles Up Her Feelings

Many of us don't want to open up about our problems because we don't want to burden others. We don't want to seem needy. I know women who don't vent to boyfriends and husbands for that very reason. They worry that their partners have too much on their own plates to have to deal with the issues of their loved ones. The problem is that we all need to be able to open up and vent. I'd argue that, as women, we are more emotional than men, and that means we probably need to even more. When we don't express ourselves, it puts our health in jeopardy.

EveryGirl Needs Someone to Talk To

Family, friends, and partners can be great sounding boards, but sometimes it's better to work things through with a therapist—

← Learning some helpful poses with Yogi Cameron.

someone who can serve as a third party and has the most open of minds to help you to assess matters clearly. Please do not see this as weakness or that there is something seriously wrong with you if you do. That's the kind of garbage thinking that oppresses us. The times I've seen a therapist, I've always felt better. In building your strong emotional foundation, it may be a good idea to meet with one—even if it's just for one session. If you're unhealthy or overweight, they may give you some insight into why, and that will only increase your chances for improvement.

Take Care of Yourself *First*

Our girls' weekend was a good reminder that first and foremost you need to take care of yourself. If you have parents, bosses, partners, and children that depend on you and whose needs you put before your own, understand that you'll be no good to any of them if you are not healthy. Make the time to eat right, exercise, and get on the fifty-year plan. And if you can't do it for yourself, then do it for those you love.

I'm asking you to step outside yourself and to try to look at your life objectively. If you're overweight, lethargic, less mobile, depressed, stressed, or, worst of all, just plain unhealthy in general, ask yourself, "Is this how I want to live the rest of my life?" Is this how you want the next fifty years to go? If you are not doing anything about it now, it's going to only get worse in the next fifty years. For me, if I'm working six to seven days a week, as I am now, and I let myself become stressed out and covered in rashes, how is that going to play out for the rest of my life? Not well. Asking myself that question has prompted me to address the issue and has inspired me to fight for solutions. Here are some ways you can do the same.

Take Responsibility

Of all the things I'm going to ask you to do, this one may be the hardest—but it is also the one that will prove to be the most valuable, not just in weight loss but also in life. Even though I don't want you to beat yourself up, I do want you to take responsibility for yourself and to own up to your shortcomings and faults. Like Jack LaLanne said, no one forced us to overeat or to be lazy.

It's hard to acknowledge the role you play in the problems or issues you have. We are all conditioned to be in denial and to blame external forces such as our upbringing, our parents, our partners, our past, or any number of people or factors. There's relief in shifting the blame—it's much more painful to blame ourselves. But not seeing how we sabotage ourselves is tantamount to treating the symptom and not the problem. Accepting our own shortcomings or issues enables us to address those problems more clearly, so that we can fix them and not repeat them.

As I said, when I started gaining weight, my aunts, uncles, and cousins made fun of me. In turn, I sat in my garage and ate gallons of ice cream—and gained a lot more weight! Whether I was rebelling against their words or soothing my pain, none of them forced that ice cream down my throat. It was my choice. Owning up to that helped me get stronger and healthier.

Attack Your Problems

Most of us don't fight for solutions. Instead, we run from our problems. We sweep them under the rug or find unhealthy distractions—such as shopping, partying, drugs (prescription or otherwise), alcohol, and, of course, food. Some people don't run. They just accept the problems and suffer through them. Or they don't treat the problem, just the symptoms. Unfortunately, I've done it, too. When

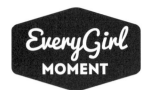

Every Girl MOMENT

When I had that stress rash I was taking steroids and applying ointments; treating the symptoms. When I altered my diet and lifestyle I treated the problem and thus cured the rash

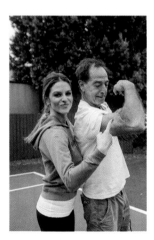

I was unhappy growing up, I would either cry in my bedroom (accept) or overeat later (escape). My cousins and I getting together for a girls' health weekend was a major step for the three of us: an example of us all finally attacking our problems.

Treat the Problem, Not the Symptom

With my dad's low blood sugar attacks, when he would teeter on death, my mom and I would take shifts monitoring him, literally twenty-four hours a day. She would never, ever sleep for fear that his sugar would drop in the night—which, at times, it did. When he was at work during the day, we would both call his bosses around the clock to make sure that he was okay. We both lived in constant fear that he would die, and I often cried myself to sleep over it. There was good reason to worry; he went comatose and was pronounced dead on more than one occasion. However, when Kev entered the picture with an outside, objective mind, things changed. He found doctors who were able to figure out why his sugar was dropping and what could be done about it. Dad got an insulin pump, which kept his blood sugar more even, and made other adjustments. Knock on wood, today he is alive and well because of it. And while I'm thankful that it all worked out, it took more than forty years of incredible anxiety and suffering for him to get there. Had we attacked the problem from the get-go, rather than the symptoms, think of what we would have been spared.

Remain in *Kaizen*

If you read my first book, you know about *kaizen*. If you didn't, *kaizen* is a Japanese philosophy that translates to remaining in a state of "continuous improvement." Always be open to new, different, and better ways of doing things, no matter how good or bad the circumstances are. I apply kaizen to all aspects of my life, from what kind of daughter I am to how I care for my dogs to how I host and report for TV to how I do the laundry to how I eat and exercise. No matter how well something seems to work, I'm open to exploring how it can be done better. It goes hand and hand with being a reporter, which is all about learning and gathering information. But you don't need to work in the news media to be always seeking new information. My parents and Kev certainly don't, and they practice kaizen. Always improving means you're always growing. And if you're not growing, you're dying. Remaining in kaizen will serve all aspects of your life, including your diet and fitness goals. No matter how good a workout routine serves me or a certain dish appeals to me, I'm always open to new ones. Whether it's a new exercise, fitness device, recipe, food, method of cooking, therapy, supplement, or remedy, I'm all ears, and you should be too!

Keep Your Mind in a State of Possibility

John Comerford is my longtime friend, acting coach, and fellow producer of AfterBuzz TV, among other projects. When he was producing and performing with me in our movie, *Adventures of Serial Buddies*, he gave a pep talk to the crew at the beginning of the shoot. I'll never forget his instructions: "*Minds must remain in the state of possibility.*" He was telling the crew to be open to possibilities rather than close-minded. In life endeavors, especially your health, keep your mind in this positive state. Don't dwell on the negative—*I'll never be in shape, I'll never quit smoking, I'll never stop overeating.* This is your mind in "impossibility,"

"Instead of obsessing over all the 'I can't' foods, focus on all the food you CAN have, the nutritious things that will fuel your body and give you the energy you need for your busy life. Your body is like a temple. Nourish it with the very best so it can keep performing for you."

–Betty Wong, editor in chief, *Fitness* magazine

and that prevents growth. Rather, consider and stay open to what *is* possible—"I may never go without sweets, but I can cut back to one day a week" or "If I switch some stuff around, maybe it is possible to get a workout in."

Nurture Healthy Relationships

As you're reading this book, notice how many times I refer to my mom, my dad, Kev, and my friends. They're a big part of how I managed to flip bad habits into good ones and how I stay on track to be healthy and fit. My father always says, "Show me who your friends are, and I'll show you who you are." This applies to personality type, integrity, and, yes, even health. If you surround yourself with people who have similar dreams and goals, you are more likely to achieve them. If you want to be healthy but are struggling to do so, hang with healthier people. And the stronger your relationships—with family, friends, coworkers, other loved ones—the healthier you are. Conversely, if you have trouble in your relationships, you're more likely to engage in unhealthy habits due to your emotional grief.

Unhealthy relationships can take many forms, whether it's people being jealous or just plain negative in your presence, or even people who engage heavily in unhealthy habits. It can be difficult to be at your healthiest when in their company—especially when you're attempting to make changes and improvements yourself. I know when I hang with people who could be described as bad influences, I will eat terribly and laugh at the very concept of working out. If I hang with healthy, active people who are forward-thinking and open-minded, I will be too.

Relationships are here to enhance our lives, not deplete them. They should "fill your cup," so to speak, not drain it. Likewise, you should provide the reverse. This doesn't mean you abandon a good friend who is sick or in need. Hell, I'd argue that helping friends when they need it *does* fill your cup. What it does mean is distancing yourself or even cutting yourself off entirely from people who use you, make you feel bad, are jealous, or don't have the best intentions for you. Being in their company will not help you to achieve the fifty-year plan.

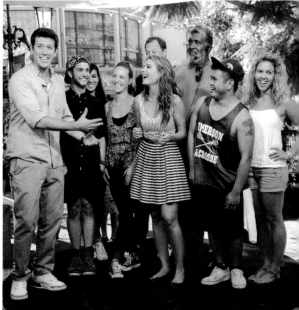

↑ Minds in possibility. We pulled off a Gangnam-style flash mob at the Grove in L.A. on *Extra* with Psy. Everyone thought it was impossible, except us!

Remain Open to New Relationships

Kev's mother, Kathie, is seventy-two years old, and since I've known her she's had close friends ranging from age twenty to ninety. And while she has friends she has known since junior high school, she has other friends she met just this year. And yes, like my dad, she looks and moves around like someone in her fifties, and again, it's not a coincidence.

My rule is, when you're young, hang out with old people. When

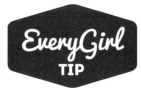

EveryGirl TIP

DON'T ENGAGE IN MENTAL VIOLENCE

When you beat yourself up and get down on yourself—including getting down on your behavior, appearance, and body—you are engaging in what Yogi Cameron calls "mental violence." You are harming yourself, and it will not help you or motivate you to get healthy—I promise.

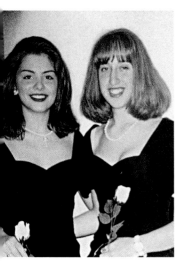

↑ Alyssa is going to hate me when she sees this! Hahaha! This is us junior year as junior marshals. We've been best friends since seventh grade.

you're old, hang out with young people. When you're in the middle, hang out with both. And have friends of as many varying backgrounds, cultures, creeds, and orientations as possible. And always, always remain open to making new ones. New relationships keep you stimulated, challenged, and spry and help you continue to flourish and grow. And what does that have to do with fitness and good health? Well, simply put, if you are not growing, you're dying—quite the opposite of good health.

Be a Good Friend . . . Especially to Yourself

Speaking of relationships and friends, you need to be a good friend to yourself! This is something I always tell Kev. If you know him, he's about the most generous friend you can have, yet, like a lot of people, he tends to beat himself up. I remind him to remember to be as good a friend to himself as he is to others. When you don't eat right or have long lapses without exercise, be a good friend to yourself and don't beat yourself up. I have spells where I neglect exercise, ignore nutrition, eat to excess, and even gain weight, like I said. However, I try not to get down on myself, and instead focus on when I can make improvements—just like any good friend would.

It's Less About Weight and More About Confidence

This is something I stressed in my previous book, but it's so worth repeating. Having confidence makes men and women more attractive. Consider sex, a subject extremely important to most men. What kind of woman do you think men are more likely to want to have sex with—one who's confident about her looks and herself or one who is insecure and embarrassed about her appearance? Get in shape for health, but whatever your weight or shape is, always be confident about yourself.

Why We Eat May Be as Important as *What* We Eat

Sometimes, it's just a matter of liking the taste of chocolate pudding. But often, it's more than that. Why do you overeat or eat mostly unhealthy foods? Are you lonely, stressed, depressed, bored? Do you just tend to crave salt? Do you merely enjoy the social aspects of eating out with friends or family?

The answers are different for everybody. I've known people who, like me, had it drilled into them as children to finish everything on their plates that they still do it today, no matter how hungry they actually are or how much food is in front of them. Sometimes people overeat just because eating is the only thing in their lives they feel they can control or their only source of comfort. Low self-esteem, perfectionism, impulsive behavior, or unhealthy relationships can also induce unhealthy eating. In extreme cases, these can be elements associated with serious eating disorders. Have an honest conversation with yourself to get at the root of any eating issues you may have. This is not about casting blame. The purpose is to help you understand the underlying reasons why you engage in unhealthy behavior so that you know how to avoid it. And as a bonus, by understanding why, you're more likely to soothe yourself with activities other than eating.

For some, again, consulting with a physician and getting a referral to a psychologist who specializes in weight loss could provide valuable answers.

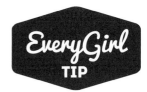

WHEN WE EAT MATTERS, TOO

Do you tend to eat when you're sad, stressed, happy, watching TV, drinking, working, driving, or even late at night? Take the time to answer this question as well as you can and then work on cutting back during those times or even switching out your comfort munchies for healthier foods.

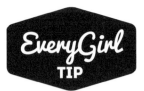

EveryGirl TIP

ASK YOURSELF: HAVE YOU EVER REGRETTED WORKING OUT?

On days his wife doesn't want to work out, my cousin Anthony will ask her: "After you're done working out, have you ever regretted it?" Sure, after a workout, you may feel tired, but you pretty much always feel good that you did it! It's a simple question, but asking it of myself has helped motivate me on days I don't feel like exercising.

Stay Young

I know this seems like a big, dumb cliché. Who doesn't want to stay young, after all? But truthfully, we can make ourselves stay young. I see it in my parents, in Kev's mom, and in people I meet every day. What I've noticed about the people who stay young is that it's mental as much as it's physical.

So how do you stay young, mentally? Most of it has been covered in the previous mantras—remaining in the state of kaizen and remaining in the state of possibility. John Comerford, who first inspired me to stay in the state of possibility, is pushing fifty yet can still do the gymnastic routine he did in high school and works circles around his twentysomething crews. It's about knowing that if you're not growing, you're dying. It's about being open to learning and to new experiences, relationships, and opportunities. It's about treating health like a marathon, not a sprint; fueling your body with quality food; and remaining active and spontaneous.

My parents have jumped onto planes to fly across the country three hours after I've gotten off the phone with them. A few years ago when I asked them to run a 5K race with me, they shrugged and said "Okay!"—even though neither of them has ever run a road race. Positivity is important, too. Aunt Flo, a surrogate aunt and friend to Kev and me, is ninety. When I saw her last month at a family party, she told me how she works out every day and then asked me to step aside so that she could get to her favorite place—the bar! Her niece Nance, also a surrogate aunt, was overweight and asthmatic her whole life, then at sixty began taking small steps—deciding to start walking instead of driving. Two years later, she does daily long-distance walks and is in great shape, and her asthma is under control! Now think of those people who move slowly, complain about aches and pains, and are negative, bitter, and closed-minded. You don't have to have reached an older age to be "old." Sadly, I know people just over thirty who are like this, and believe it or not, it shows on their face and in their posture. It's sad and prohibitive to good health, but it's something I think can be avoided with the right outlook and attitude. Staying young mentally means that the physical portion—eating right and exercising—will come more easily.

Bring a Sense of Urgency . . . to Everything You Do

Here's another good way to stay young and fit—carry a sense of urgency throughout your day. Addressing problems and completing tasks immediately ensures general overall success in business and in personal matters. For example, there's a tremendous sense of urgency at my office. We're constantly shooting out e-mails, crossing tasks off our lists, and just plain "getting shit done." With a sense of urgency, we move about so rapidly that we're always in motion and burning calories. Since a body in motion stays in motion, I'm always more motivated to exercise after work. And by acting with urgency, I get so many tasks completed that I can more easily free myself up to work out or even just enjoy downtime cuddling with my dogs and watching Netflix.

Break from "Convenience Conditioning"

As Americans we choose the most convenient or easiest option in everything we do. When offered elevators, escalators, the parking space near the mall entrance, or shortcuts of all kinds, we

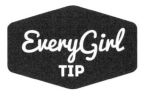

EASY NOW, HARD LATER

Kev's father died a couple of years before I met Kev, but hearing about him, I regret never getting to know him. Kev says that one of his dad's favorite sayings was "Easy now, hard later . . . . Hard now, easy later." He'd say these few simple words in a singsong way when Kev and his brothers would complain about doing work. It's as great a mantra for working toward your health goals as it is for working toward your dreams and attaining success. Eat right and exercise now, and you'll have it easier later. Eat poorly and be sedentary, and you'll definitely have it harder later.

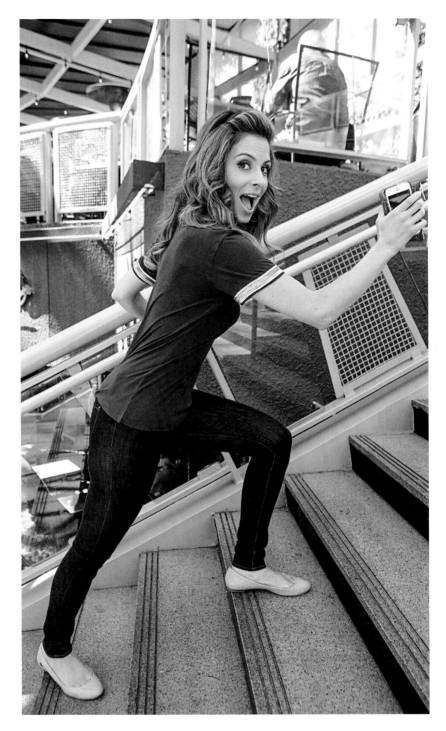

instinctively choose the fastest, easiest, and most convenient options. For the purposes of health and staying fit, I consciously seek to do the opposite.

I do things like walk instead of drive or climb stairs instead of taking escalators. I've trained myself to resist taking the most convenient option in my daily activities to taking the more physically demanding ones.

As you move forward, when engaging in daily activities of your own, don't always opt for the most convenient way, opt for the one that involves the most exercise and burns the most calories.

Don't Set Yourself Up for Failure

At one point Kev was battling depression and trying to get back on his feet, I asked him to try surfing with me. He said he'd watch me but refused to try it himself. When I asked him why, he had an interesting response. He said that to break his depression, he needed to take baby steps. He was putting his energy into things he knew he could accomplish rather than taking steps or attempting tasks that he knew he couldn't. Surfing, for example, is tough to pick up; he felt that trying to do it and not succeeding would only exacerbate his depression.

The same philosophy can be applied to any diet or fitness goal. By trying to take steps that are too big, trying to do a 180-degree turnaround, you could very well be setting yourself up for the same kind of failure. Extreme workouts out of the gate may leave you too sore to want to work out ever again! Or they might seem so difficult that your self-esteem takes a hit, discouraging you. When it comes to diet and fitness, engage in little tasks that you know you can achieve—small steps, a few degrees at a time.

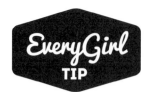

OUR LIVES ARE GARDENS—ALWAYS WORKS IN PROGRESS

For gardens to prosper, they must be continually hoed and tilled. Weeds must be removed, flowers must be clipped, crops must be picked, soil must be turned over if the garden is to be a healthy one. The same goes for our lives. We must be constantly turning over and hoeing the soil for our lives to be healthy—making changes and adjustments in all areas.

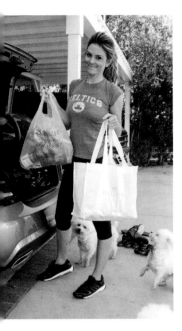

PHYSICAL FOUNDATION

D.O.C.—Declutter, Organize, Clean!

What does organizing your closet, washing the dirty dishes in your sink, and throwing out the stacks of magazines that have been sitting on your coffee table or nightstand for the past year have to do with losing weight? A lot more than you might think. I've seen people perpetually depressed, moody, negative, overwhelmed, stressed out and exhausted but never knew *why*. Well, when I saw the cluttered and messy environments in which they live, sleep, drive, and work, I knew the reason!

Chaotic, dark, and depressing environments are not positive places to relax, recover, and recharge in. They don't create a healthy mind-set or motivate a person to exercise, eat properly, and make healthy choices. Think about it: When we're depressed, the first thing most of us do is eat. When your own home isn't conducive to R&R, you're going to be tired and thus crave and consume unhealthy foods.

I understand that many of you may think I'm crazy, but trust me. I used to be sloppy and didn't realize how much it affected my health and the way I felt until I addressed it.

Declutter!

By decluttering your home, car, desk, drawers, wallet, computers, work areas, and life, you will feel better right out of the gate, I promise you. It will be as though a huge weight has been lifted from your shoulders; the two bags of bricks you've been carrying around have finally been set down. And guess what? Those healthy feelings will strengthen your emotional foundation. It's so much easier to work out and eat properly—not to mention be more effective in other areas of your life—when you've cleared out the clutter.

Studies show that physical clutter competes for your mind's attention and overloads your senses, decreasing performance, increasing stress, and impairing your ability to think. Similar studies indicate that ridding yourself of clutter actually releases the same pleasant endorphins in your brain that people experience when they exercise, otherwise known as the runner's high. In feng shui, an ancient Chinese wisdom that shows you how to balance the energies of physical environments to assure positive health, fortune, and well-being, clutter is associated with blocked *chi* or blocked energy. According to feng shui, letting go of clutter will get your energy flowing.

My mom was, and still can be, a pack rat and guess what, so am I! Being on television, I get so many items sent to me that my house, office, and car are constantly filling up with boxes and boxes of things. I know, poor me, right? But seriously, because I grew up poor, I want to hang onto absolutely everything. I guess I think it

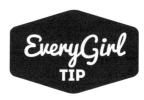

SAY GOODBYE TO KNICK-KNACKS!

Simplify your decor and free yourself of all those dust-collecting knick-knacks. And don't rationalize it with the argument of "this is my style." Your style is hurting you, keeping you from getting ahead in life, feeling great, and being happy. Just try it. Keep tabletops and desks as sparse and as free of objects as possible. It will go a long way to positive mental health, and that will help you achieve better physical health.

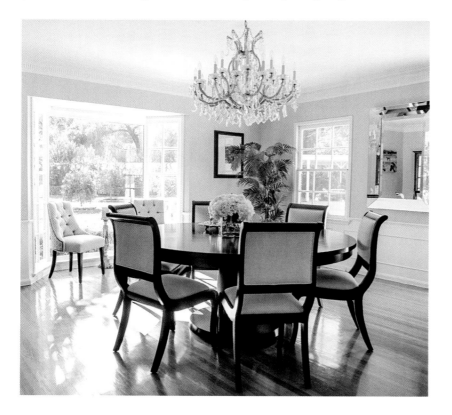

will make me feel happier or more secure. Yet it's only when I take the time to give the stuff away and get it all out of my office, car, and house that I actually feel good. And truth be told, I feel amazing afterward, completely energized and ready to take on the world—which includes working out. But don't just take it from me. Check out any Apple store, the public face of one of the world's most successful chains and brands, and notice how bright, clean, and simple the decor is and how positive the staff is. None of it is a coincidence. The late, great Steve Jobs spent years testing the right layout for stores and concluded that they needed to be as clutter-free as possible, because clutter equals an unpleasant, negative, and stressful environment that is not conducive to work or purchasing!

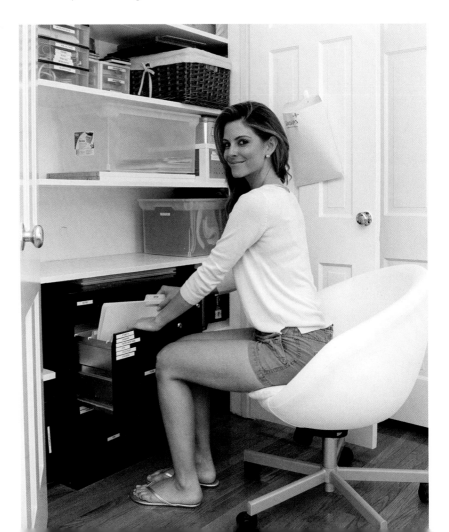

MY EVERYGIRL SLOB JOURNEY

Just recently, my office slowly and quietly transformed into a storage room. Mail and packages would simply get dropped inside. Working such long days, I never had time to even go in there to work, and as the weeks turned to months, it got out of hand. On my one day off, even though I was exhausted, I took action and got rid of it all. I cleaned out all of my old outdated and unnecessary files, got rid of all the old furniture, and started fresh. I went to Ikea and spent a few hundred dollars on a new desk and some cabinets and painted the walls. I threw out two huge trash bags of junk. Even though I was tired, I ended up getting a wonderful burst of energy from doing it.

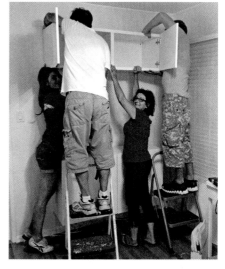

When the room was clean with simple decor, I had another realization. It wasn't that I didn't have time to go into my office, as I had initially suspected, it was more that I had actually dreaded going in there. With all of the junk out and the new makeover, I am now sooooooo much happier and so much more productive.

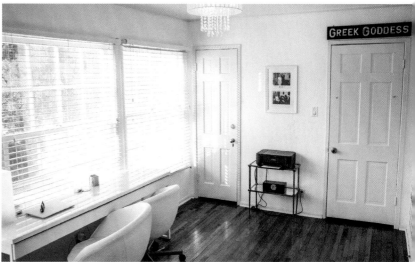

P.S.: The new office was so inspiring and uplifting, it's where I wrote much of this book! You just can't underestimate how much a cluttered and disorganized environment can drag you down until you take the steps to fix it.

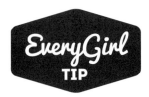

EveryGirl TIP

INSPIRATION BOARDS
I create inspiration boards all the time to help me visualize success goals, including those for diet and fitness. I cut out pictures of things I want to have, places I want to be or places that create a calm or happy feeling, plus images and quotes that inspire me; and I paste them to a large whiteboard. I hang my inspiration boards in my office or even put them next to my bed. They always help me reach my goals.

Get Organized!

The same benefits come from being organized—hanging up clothes rather than just throwing them on the floor, filing things properly rather than having them pile up on your desk (remember: file, don't pile!), or just putting items back in their proper places in general. It takes far less time to do those things than it does to scramble to find things later and avoid more stress and chaos.

Be Clean!

Besides being clutter-free and organized, you also want a clean environment free of dust, dirt, and garbage. Don't you always feel better after a shower? You'll feel better in your environment if it's clean, too. The better you feel, the healthier you'll behave.

Again, as a reformed slob I still have my moments where I get lazy and leave dirty dishes in my sink or garbage in my car. And guess what, it never feels good when I do. Rather, when things are wiped down, vacuumed, and polished I feel great and more ready to engage in life's healthier pursuits.

See Your Home as Your Sanctuary

I encourage you to declutter, clean, and organize your home, car, and work area because these are the places that most of us spend the majority of our time. I especially ask you to concentrate most on the place you live—whether it's a bedroom in your parents' house, an apartment, or a house. Though I believe getting fit and healthy is all about being active and urgent, you will need your downtime. Your living space is where you start and end your days, and it's crucial you feel your best when you do. As I said in *The EveryGirl's Guide to Life*, the good news is that you don't need a Ph.D. to declutter, organize, and clean. You just need to invest some time—a weekend or a few vacation days. After that, it's routine maintenance. Later you'll read that I'm against 180 degree turnarounds or extreme life changes, but when it comes to organizing and decluttering, I'm all for an about-face. Suck it up, invest the time, and get it done. The energy you invest in this will be well worth it in the long run. Good things will come soon after, I promise.

Take Your Inventory

Now we shift from your physical environment to the physical you! In keeping with our "Health first" mantra, as much as it's important to get in shape, it's more important to get a complete look at your health picture, whether it's blood pressure, cholesterol, blood sugar, thyroid, vitamin D, or other issues. I don't obsess over visiting multiple doctors. If something's wrong, yes, I listen to my body, but I try not to overanalyze what's going on. Besides annual gynecological visits, I have an annual physical around the new year—scheduling it then makes it easier to remember. I think it's important for all women to be tested and checked annually, including having blood work done. I think it's also important to know and be aware of any relevant family medical history.

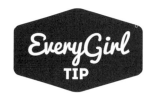

LESS DECOR IS MORE—
And more affordable, too! Keep it simple and use sound and color to enhance your mood. Small fountains with a trickle of running water, for example, offer a nice relaxing touch to an environment as do pleasant aromas. I especially love scented candles.

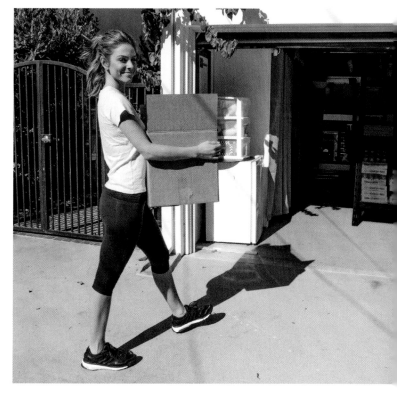

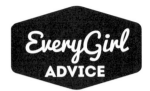

EveryGirl ADVICE

LACK OF SLEEP AGES YOU

Sleep is when our bodies truly rejuvenate, but in case you're still not motivated to get proper sleep, keep in mind that lack of sleep prematurely ages you. Research shows that women who skimp on sleep are twice as likely to have fine lines, uneven skin tone, and other signs of aging. Plus their skin takes longer to recover from sun damage.

Don't Rush to Take Pills

If the results of your test show that something is low or high, I want to caution you against just taking a pill or medicine to help it get to normal levels. I'd prefer you to do some research and talk in depth with the doctor about the medication and the issue to see if there are any lifestyle changes that can help as well, or even possibly replace the medication. In some cases, the fix will be dietary. Shifting the way you eat has a profound impact on all the important chemical reactions in your body. Remember to treat the problem, not the symptom.

When I had that stress rash, I rushed to treat it with steroid creams and pills. The rash would subside temporarily, only to return in a fiercer form. When I met with Yogi Cameron, he assessed my emotional foundation and helped me figure out what I needed to do to curb my stress. Next he assessed my physical foundation and what I was eating. At the time, I was loading up on hot, spicy foods as well as candy and other processed foods. These are what Cameron calls "heating foods." In essence, they physically heat your body up. In my case, eating those energetic foods ended up igniting my rashes. By consuming unprocessed "cooling" foods and managing my stress, the rash eventually calmed down and subsided. The experience served as a fine example of treating the problem, not the symptom; how shifting the way you eat can profoundly affect your health, and why you shouldn't simply and solely rely on medicine.

Sleep Helps Your Diet

I'm convinced that there has been no time in history when Americans have been so busy, been spread so thin, moved so quickly. We're pulled in so many directions—work, family, friends, obligations—that few of us get our necessary seven to eight hours of sleep. When we're tired we usually choose sugary foods, which leads to a zap of energy and then a crash, followed by the need for more sugar. Not only that, but scientists show that people who don't get enough sleep have more of the hormones that trigger hunger and less of the hormones that make you feel full.

Sleep Is the Best Medicine

Whether you are nursing an injury, recovering from an operation or battling a flu, virus, or cold, you'll heal faster with some good, old-fashioned sleep! When the body sleeps, it's exerting the least amount of energy, allowing the greatest amount of healing to occur. So whether it's a cold or a twisted ankle, catch as many Zs as you can.

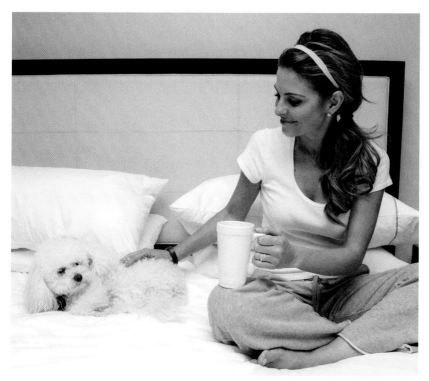

EASY WAYS TO GET YOUR Zs

→ **Don't leave your phone by your bed**. *If you do, shut off the ringer.*

→ **A cool, dark room makes for the best sleep environment**. *Invest in good sheets and a comforter and keep the thermostat low even during winter. I found amazing sheets for thirty bucks at a store called Tuesday Morning.*

→ **Wind down before bed** *with decaf tea or hot water or a warm bath with Epsom salts. If you exercise or watch TV before bed, it may be too stimulating and you could have trouble falling asleep.*

→ **Avoid caffeine** *for three hours before you go to bed.*

→ **No eating before bed,** *either. It's unhealthy for many reasons. First, your body will be busy digesting your food and that prevents you from getting deep sleep. Second—it's not like you're burning the calories off while you're lying there. Eating before bed can lead to weight gain.*

→ **Don't work in bed**. *Again, it's too much stimulation on your mind and prevents deep sleep. When I do, I know I don't get the best sleep.*

→ **Use white noise.** *I use a small fan to drown out other noises and lull myself to sleep. There are also plenty of smartphone apps that can simulate any noise you like—fans, the ocean, trains, thunder. There are also great meditation apps that I use as well. All can have the same effect—helping to create a quality sleep environment. On my iPhone I have an app called "White Noise."*

→ **If you go to bed listening to the radio or watching TV, set a timer** *so that it shuts off after you're asleep.*

In my office and on my nightstand I keep an eye mask that has speakers built into it. It's called the Remedy Heat Sensitive Memory Foam Sleep Mask, and I bought it on amazon.com. Using it, listening to my white noise app, helps me sneak in those ten minute naps when I need them.

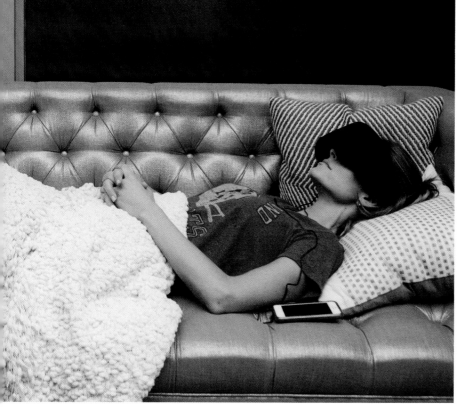

Maria's 10-Minute Nap

Recently, I went through a stretch where I was getting only between four and five hours of sleep a night due to work. I compensated for it with periodic 10-minute naps, and they really helped. The naps allowed me to recharge and refocus. One time, I was so tired that I set out to take a 10-minute nap at 6 p.m. and didn't wake up until 7 the next morning! Clearly, my body needed that. And though the 10-minute nap can work temporarily, be sure to remain mindful of your body's long-term needs, too.

Listen to Your Body!

As much as I want you to act with urgency and stay in motion, you have to learn to listen to your body. If you're tired, then sleep. If you're injured, then allow yourself time to heal. If your body needs

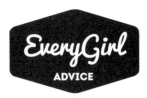

When Kev gets a cold or any kind of illness or is just plain wiped out, he'll say he needs to "tap out." If you are a fan of ultimate fighting, you know that when a fighter "taps out," he's physically tapping the ring apron—signaling to the referee that he's surrendering. When Kev's says he's tapping out, he means he's quitting work or whatever else he's doing to hit the sheets and sleep the illness or exhaustion off. I'm the worst when it comes to tapping out. I'll get sick and then continue to push through with my work only to extend the length of the illness, whereas Kev is done with his cold or flu in less than forty-eight hours. I'll also work past exhaustion and thus risk lowering my immunity and getting sick.

This goes for injuries, too. If you are feeling body aches and strains while working out, then simply stop what you're doing. If you are hobbled with an injury, allow yourself time to heal properly. The bottom line is, don't be afraid to tap out the next time you're wiped out, sick, or injured. You'll be better off in the long run.

hydration or food, then get it what it needs. If it needs a vacation or escape, then get it that, too. As you get healthier, your body will send you clearer signals about what it needs. Be alert and open to hearing those signals and then be sure to listen when you receive them.

Invest in Your Health

While the core of my being is to have EveryGirl save as much money as possible, I also said health *is* the most important thing in life, remember? Therefore, you can't put a price on it, and sometimes you can't always do it for less. Some of you will be able to exercise at the foot of your bed with twenty dollars' worth of equipment and take five dollars' worth of Tupperware veggies to work for lunch. However, some people may need trainers, gyms, expensive equipment, prepared meals, and other things that cost money. And if that's what it's gonna take to get you on the road to better health and the fifty-year plan, then invest the money to do so.

After ten years of working out on a Bowflex, Kev claimed he needed new equipment to motivate him. He wanted to change things up and do some free weights along with his usual resistance training. Sure enough, he bought a new Powertec machine for about eight hundred dollars. I rolled my eyes and thought he was just making excuses and wasting his money. But I was wrong. As of 2014, Kev has been at it for two years, hasn't missed a single workout, and has had great results.

The point, though, isn't for you to buy a Bowflex or a Powertec. The point is, don't be afraid to invest in anything that will help you achieve your diet and fitness goals.

Open Your Mind to New Challenges

Ask yourself, what have you always wanted to do that you never felt confident or able to do? Maybe run a 5K or a marathon.

Maybe go for a weekend hike in the mountains with your family. Maybe learn to ski or paddle board. As long as it's not super extreme or something that will break your spirit should you fail, then by all means step out of your comfort zone and try it. When Kev refused to try surfing due to his depression, he was also lifting weights and running on the treadmill in an effort to recover, so I knew he didn't need to be pushed further. For *Dancing with the Stars*, I was resistant and terrified, but I opened my mind to the new challenge and was rewarded in the process

↓ I know if I had allowed myself a little time to heal and rest during *DWTS*, I would have been better at each dance. I saw proof with my final tango. I rested the day before our encore, and I was a million times better. Listen to your body!

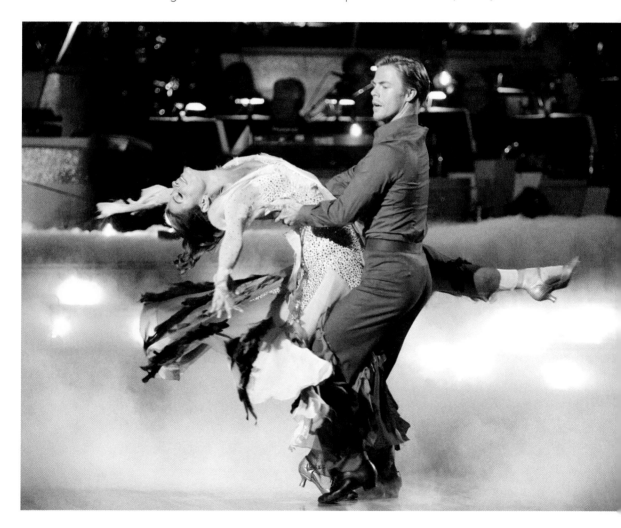

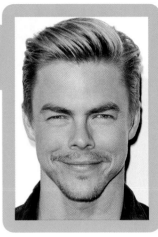

MARIA TALKS WITH ... DEREK HOUGH

What makes a woman attractive?

For me, the look is important, but it's also about the health aspect. Someone who's fit, who can go for a jog or a hike and keep up with an adventurous type of lifestyle, which I like. I'm a very physical, active person. You'll get an athletic body as a result of that lifestyle, versus someone who sits at home and doesn't do anything. Whatever body you happen to get through doing those types of things will be your natural body type, I suppose. I think also, especially butts. I love butts. Too skinny is never a good thing.

What do you think makes a women sexy?

Someone who loves adventure and being spontaneous and living life. Physically, I don't know. I feel like you can look sexy in sweats.

You've danced with so many women on *Dancing with the Stars*, and some of them have trimmed down and lost weight during the process. What's the biggest change you've noticed in them?

It goes back to energy levels, that's what I've noticed in that aspect. But what I notice more than anything is the self-confidence, and I think it's a domino effect. I think that since "self-discipline" sounds like such a negative thing, it has such a negative association. Or even "sacrifice"; you're sacrificing your time to do something. But sacrifice is such a positive thing. For instance, if somebody says they're dieting and that they have to sacrifice chocolate, that has such a negative association. But what sacrifice means is giving up something good for something better. It means you're giving up chocolate because you want to feel better and have more energy, you give up sugar because you want to lose a little weight. So, DWTS participants give up something good for something better.

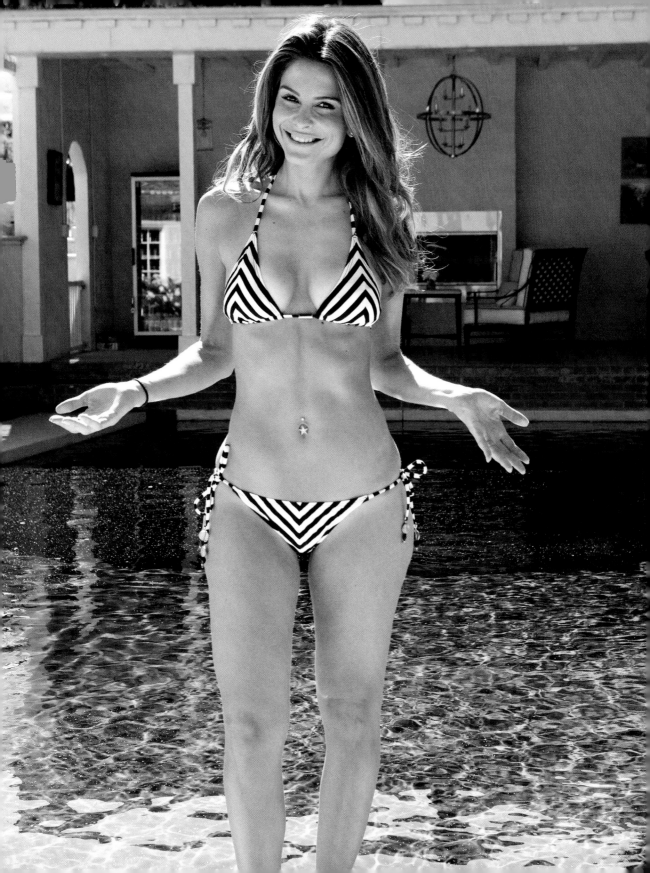

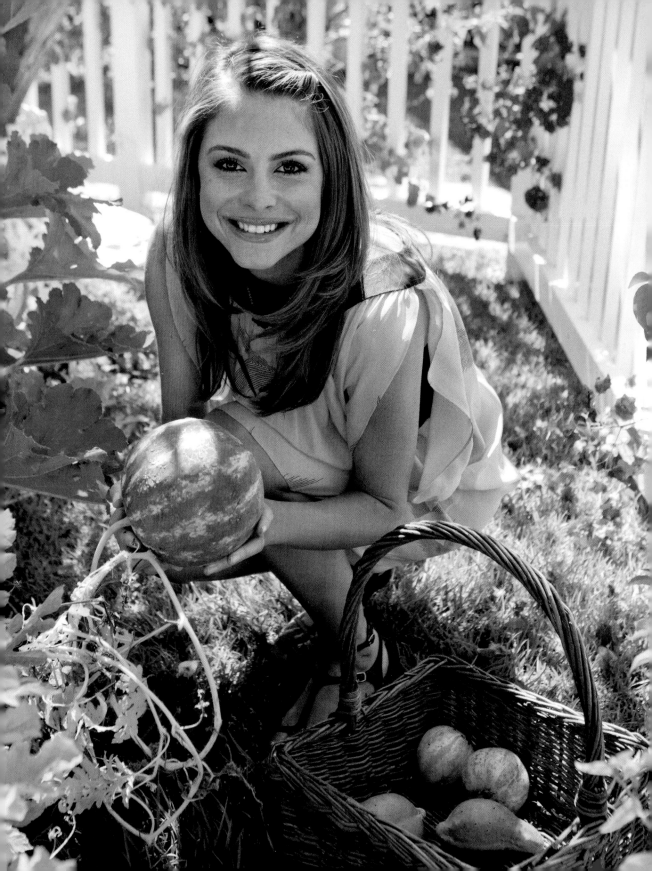

Chapter 4

EveryGirl's Eleven Diet and Fitness Rules to Live By

By now you probably want to jump into the more concrete steps to weight loss and fitness—what foods to eat and what exercises to do. But remember the point of the book: to achieve success in diet, fitness, and overall health for the next 50-plus years. While I believe it's not as hard to achieve as one might think, it's a battle nonetheless, and I want to arm you with enough ammunition as possible. Therefore, before we get to those concrete steps, I'm going to share, and in some cases, reiterate, every pearl of wisdom I can to help ensure your success. On that note, here are eleven rules EveryGirl should keep in mind.

Being Healthy Is More Important Than Being Thin

Let's face it, the entire diet industry as well as the messages we get from Hollywood, the media, and pretty much our entire country revolve around weight and size. Lose more pounds. Fit into smaller clothes. Get thin! I understand how and why EveryGirl would be motivated to lose pounds and inches and reduce her dress size. I admit that I really enjoy being in shape. And considering the obesity epidemic that we're in, there's absolutely nothing wrong with trying to lose weight. The main thing I want to convey, though, is that thin cannot compete with healthy. *Health* is *the* most important thing in your life.

Many of us take health for granted and tend to think that living the good life, being wealthy, or being thin are the most important things. It's only when we lose our health that we realize how wrong we were. I was thin when I almost died in that hospital in France.

Nobody is more proud of my success than my father. Often, he'll say that he never imagined anything like it in his entire lifetime. Just as often, he reminds me how appreciative I need to be of my success, how little I should complain, and how hard I should work to maintain it.

But if it gets to the point where the stress, my eating habits, and the pressure of my schedule start to compromise my health, that's where he draws the line. No matter how proud he is of my success, he'd rather see me quit and lose it all than to lose my good health. More than once he has told Kev and me to slow down, emphatically stating in his thick Greek accent that "The most important thing is your health—period!" As a type 1 diabetic who has literally been pronounced dead due to low-blood-sugar comas on umpteen occasions, he has a deeper appreciation of this than most people. But this is a message I've consistently heard from other successful and wise people who have either lost loved ones to poor health or have experienced poor health themselves.

Hey, if you can be healthy and thin (and, of course, I am going to show you how to do that!), then more power to you, but risking everything to be thin is not worth it and makes no sense in the big picture. I know more than a few thin people who are unhealthy. They smoke cigarettes, starve themselves, live on gallons of diet soda and energy drinks, or use drugs or other such unhealthy means to stay thin. As a result, some of them will not live long lives, and those who do may not live *quality* lives. Many, if not most, are also unhappy. I go back to my father, who in retirement can enjoy life to the fullest because his primary goal was good health. That goal naturally resulted in his being trim, as it will you.

EVERYGIRL RULE 2
Know the Skinny Truth

Thank you, Kim Kardashian (a close friend I'm blessed to have in my life), for exposing what Kev and most of my guy friends have been screaming for years. The "skinny truth" is that guys like a girl with curves! As Kev always says, having curves is what makes us girls. He fell for me when I was forty pounds heavier and often says that

"Losing weight is not about being on a diet or a detox or fast. It's about a decision you make to be healthy for the rest of your life."
—Lucy Danziger, editor-in-chief, *Self* magazine

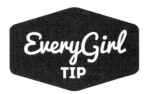

**THE SKINNY
ON WRINKLES**

If I haven't convinced you
that you don't need to be
thin as a rail for health
reasons, then consider the
fact that when you're skinny,
the wrinkles on your face
show more because you lack
the fat on your face
to fill them out!

he misses those extra pounds. My *Extra* co-host, Mario Lopez, concurs that girls with curves catch his eye more often, too. I'm sure there are guys who dig skinny girls, but for the most part the "waif look" is a creation of the media—not real men and women.

Like I said, we are driven by the media. Whether we're talking about fashion, style, or even body type, the media truly dictates what's desirable. We see the skinniest of models on the runways and on magazine covers and instantly think we need that kind of body, too. It's no different than seeing a new hairstyle or cut of jeans. When we see things in bright lights or are told by Hollywood or the media that we must have them, our knee-jerk response is to believe them.

But consider the real reason most photographers and designers put super-skinny models on display. It's mainly because that's *their* personal preference. They personally prefer to photograph or to see their clothing worn by über-skinny models, and that preference gets passed on to us. If you poll the guys you know and ask them what *they* would prefer, you'll get the real skinny.

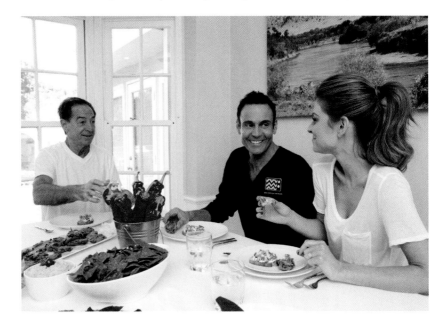

EVERYGIRL RULE 3
It's a Marathon, Not a Sprint

When I was forty pounds heavier and decided to lose the weight, I took a long-term, gradual approach. I didn't have the willpower to go on an extreme diet and drop all the foods I loved. And with work, paying bills, my family and friends, and my relationship with Kev, I certainly didn't have the time

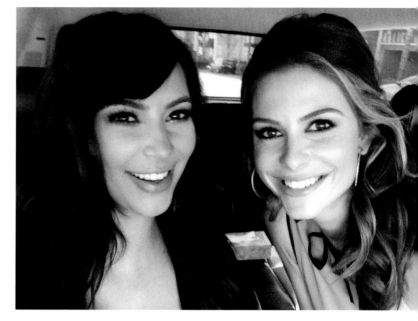

to exercise two hours a day. It took a year or so, but I lost the forty pounds. Little did I know that slow and steady was not only the most realistic way to lose weight but also the smartest. It's the main reason I never gained the weight back.

But again it's not just about keeping the weight off, it's about being healthy for the duration of your life. And once again, I use my dad as a shining example of someone who has taken the marathon approach via eating well and being active for the past forty-five years.

The long-term approach is also the most logical one. Let's face it—life in general is a marathon, not a sprint. Most of us are gonna be here for a long time—longer on average than any generation before us. Therefore, we need to address diet and fitness with that fact in mind, the way my father has. The good news is that marathons are run slowly. The changes you make in your lifestyle can be slow and gradual and still get you where you want to go!

↑ A pregnant Kim Kardashian and me on our way to lunch in Beverly Hills. It really upset me that people were so cruel to her during her pregnancy. We should be lifting each other up, not tearing each other down.

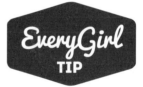

AVOID CRASH DIETING
Short-term crash diets often slow your metabolism, so that when you return to eating normally you'll gain weight back faster. Worse your body instinctively puts on extra pounds as a kind of insurance in case you're foolish enough to attempt another crash diet down the road.

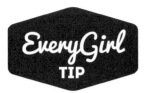

EveryGirl TIP

IT TAKES 21 DAYS TO BREAK A BAD HABIT

Many of the health and diet experts I know say that it takes about three weeks for you to change a behavior and form a new habit. So there's a challenge for you: Can you make it three weeks without your old vice and replace it with a healthier substitute? If you can, you have a much greater chance of getting the body you want.

EVERYGIRL RULE 4
Don't Attempt a 180

Here's a mistake I see EveryGirl make time and time again. We're upset with the way our bodies look, and we swear it's time to make a change. However, instead of making one change, we make a million changes. We do a complete 180-degree turnaround. In most cases, those changes are so enormous, drastic, and overwhelming that we can't possibly stick with them. Or we don't see results fast enough and get discouraged. And even if we can maintain all those changes long enough to get in shape, sooner or later it all gets to be too much. We resume our old habits and we gain the weight back—and then some.

Why does the 180 approach generally fail? Because it's incredibly hard to change everything about the way you eat and exercise overnight. We still have jobs, pressures, stresses, a social life, and so many other factors that make it virtually impossible to overhaul everything.

In my personal quest for a better body and health, I finally succeeded when I eased out of old habits and into new ones. Change—and I mean, sustainable change—takes time. Yes, I want you to make changes, but I want you to be realistic about what you can do, and I want to give you the best shot at overall success.

I think you will find that a lot of the changes I suggest in the eating and exercise chapters of this book will be fairly easy to do. But I also know that every woman is different. Let's say you have a two-decade-old diet soda habit that you've decided you want to kick. You might not want to tackle that challenge at the same time you're starting a workout routine or shifting the way you think about your meals. Instead of a 180-degree approach, start with 10 or 15 or 20 degrees and just inch it closer and closer to 180. So when you get close to facing the opposite direction—the point

THE EVERYGIRL'S GUIDE TO DIET AND FITNESS

where you look, feel, and really are healthy and happy—those changes will simply part of your lifestyle and be permanent.

EVERYGIRL RULE 5
Avoid Being Rigid!

For my online talk show *Conversations with Maria Menounos,* I conduct hour-long, one-on-one, sit-down interviews with stars and powerful people. It's in these interviews (and the ones I've done previously in my career) that I've received so much useful information. In one particular interview I did with Perez Hilton I learned about his own amazing weight-loss and fitness journey. He was once overweight but today rocks some serious abs and even launched *FitPerez.com,* a site dedicated to fitness. In the last part of our interview, I asked Perez what general advice he would give to others. He said "Don't be too rigid." If you are not flexible in your attitude and actions, you'll stunt your growth. While this applies to all aspects of life, Perez specifically mentioned how important it is when it comes to fitness. For example, he didn't just stick to one

↓ On the set of *Conversations with Maria* with a very fit Perez.

form of exercise, such as just lifting weights to firm and build his muscles. He applied yoga to stretch, cardio to sweat, and a whole host of other activities. He wasn't and still isn't afraid to try new means and methods. Case in point: He literally "hopped" to our interview on a pair of new spring-loaded exercise boots, designed to put less impact on your joints when you're jogging (and have fun in the process).

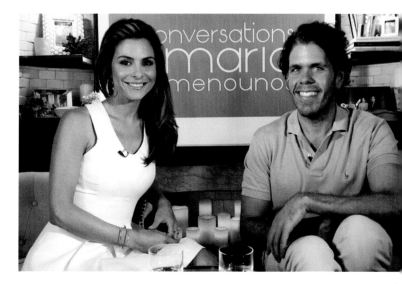

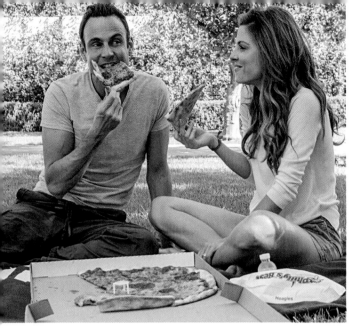

You can read more about Perez's insights on page 84.

Being rigid or strictly adhering to a regimented diet and workout plan only puts more pressure on you. When you happen to cheat or miss a workout, you get discouraged. Discouragement is exactly what you shouldn't be feeling—especially when you're trying to make changes and improvements. And in terms of weight loss, toning, and building muscles, the best results come when you continually change up your fitness routine.

But you do need some structure. With too much wiggle room, there's too much space for error and too much of a chance that you'll overindulge or never get on track at all.

So how do you find a sense of flexibility in a diet plan without being so loose that you don't do anything at all? You build a fence. It's a great parenting analogy. To raise healthy, independent kids, you give them boundaries but let them roam within those boundaries. If you don't let kids off the metaphorical porch, they'll either stay on that porch and stunt their growth, or they'll get so stir-crazy and restricted that they will be looking for ways to bust loose, wander off into the woods, and end up in a lot of trouble. So you put up a fence, but you give them freedom to explore within the boundaries of your "yard." And if all goes right, you've set up a set of rules with some flexibility in them. And if my parenting analogy doesn't hit home, then think about an artist and a painting. The artist has the freedom to do whatever he wants on the canvas—yet the painting still has a canvas size and frame to contain it.

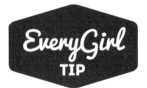

MODEL INSPIRATION

I'm not the only one in Hollywood who eats things like pizza and French fries. Many of my fit friends in Hollywood do, too. Chrissy Teigen is a top *Sports Illustrated* swimsuit model who is as fun and laid back as you can get. When we're out together she's not nibbling on lettuce. She'll order a burger and fries or whatever she craves. The thing is she may not, or does not feel the need to, eat every last morsel on the plate. It's all about portion control and moderation.

I haven't cut pizza and dessert out of my diet. I eat them, but within the limits I've set for myself. I don't eat them every day, and I don't have half a cake or an entire pizza in one sitting (the way I used to when I was in college). And if I have pizza, I may not have dessert on the same day. This approach is far less rigid and because of that I'm far less likely to rebel.

In part 2 of this book I'm going to build you a fence, but you, as an EveryGirl, have to have some room to wander, to explore what works for you and to occasionally give in to temptation without getting lost in the woods. As you'll see when I detail my own habits, I, too, have a hard time eating the same way all the time and exercising.

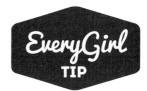

**RUN YOUR BODY ON
HIGH-QUALITY FUEL**

If you put low-grade fuel in your car, the result is a car that runs like crap, with a shortened life expectancy. Put high-grade quality fuel in your car and the result is a car that runs well and lasts longer. The same can be said for your body, as is shown by people like my father. Give your body quality fuel—food that comes from the ground—and you'll get the same results! Not processed food. Real food.

EVERYGIRL RULE 6
Eat Food That Comes from the Ground

Though I strayed from this rule in college, I mainly ate fresh fruits, whole grains, and vegetables growing up. But I never knew just how important that was to health until I was introduced to Yogi Cameron. Through the experience with my rash and subsequent other medical issues, Cameron proved to me just how much the food we consume affects our overall health and well-being. When I asked Cameron for a list of the best foods to eat. His answer turned out to be the number one tip for dietary health. He smiled and said, "Just try your best to eat food that comes from the ground and you'll be fine."

When you opt for foods that come from the ground over processed ones, you will also avoid the energy fluctuations that cause so many of us to reach for the instant pick-me-up junk foods that inevitably lead to bigger crashes—and then leave you reaching for even more junk to give yourself a boost. Real foods will provide you with sustainable energy and contain

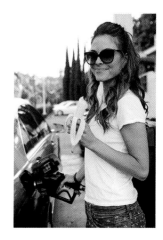

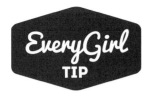

RECOMMENDED READING
I love Yogi Cameron's books, *The Guru in You* and *The One Plan.* I highly suggest them.

the vitamins, minerals, fiber, and antioxidants that your body needs to get and stay healthy, inside and out. They're also a whole lot less fattening.

EVERYGIRL RULE 7
Drink (Hot) Water for Weight Loss

When it comes to dieting, there's no magic solution. But there is such a thing as a secret weapon: water. Experts suggest that you drink eight to ten glasses a day. It hydrates, detoxes, and cleanses your body; it's good for your skin; and it fills you up and curbs your appetite. Often when we think we are hungry, we are actually just dehydrated. However, I take what the experts say and go one step further: I don't just drink water. I drink hot water.

As I give you the details of my diet plan, I will make many suggestions, but drinking hot water is one of the things I suggest up front. Yogi Cameron taught me that hot water can give you all the benefits of drinking water, but if you drink it after a meal, it helps with digestion. Think of it as melting the food in your stomach. It also has wonderful psychological and practical advantages. It's warm and comforting, like coffee, but cleaner. Because you're sipping it throughout the day, it helps your stomach stay satisfied. And, to speak even more practically, it gives your hands and mouth something to do—which is one of the reasons so many of us reach for bad foods, especially when we're stressed or crazy.

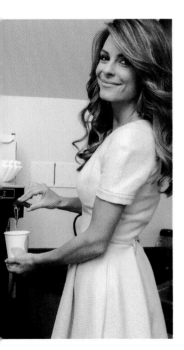

I keep an electric kettle at my home and office. Every morning, I fill a travel mug with hot water and sip it while I drive to work. Then I keep refilling it throughout the day. It's better than a caffeinated or chemically processed diet beverage, and it helps me cope with stress and keeps me from reaching for junk. You can squeeze a fresh lemon in for flavor (or even other fruits as a way

THE EVERYGIRL'S GUIDE TO DIET AND FITNESS

to mix things up), which also aids in digestion and is further detoxifying. But having to buy, cut, and pack lemons may not be convenient. Often enough, I drink my hot water straight.

In a way, drinking hot water is probably the simplest—yet most powerful—dieting strategy of all. When Keven had a stomach infection, he drank plain hot water until the infection subsided. He enjoyed drinking hot water and kept the habit going. It curbed his appetite and in the following months he lost twenty pounds. Though I luckily never gained that first forty pounds back, I do gain and lose a few pounds here and there. When Yogi Cameron put me on the hot water plan, I lost ten pounds myself. Truthfully, Kev and I didn't know weight loss would be a benefit of drinking hot water, it just happened naturally; and I've been spreading the word ever since.

EVERYGIRL RULE 8
ABM—Always Be Moving

A few months ago, my schedule was completely crazy, and I noticed that my jeans were a little tight and that my other clothes weren't fitting the way they used to. I stepped on the scale, and sure enough, I had gained a little weight. I wondered what had happened. My eating hadn't changed. But then I realized: My activity level *had* changed. Because my schedule was so jammed, at *Extra* I was riding the golf cart back and forth between shots rather than walking from point A to point B like I used to. I skimped on my quickie five-minute stairs workouts, and I had slowed down my daily physical activity. Add to that the fact that I don't consistently do official twenty-minute daily, or even weekly, workout routines. It all caught up with me. Once I realized that, I was reminded to adhere to one of my daily mantras from the past: ABM, or Always Be Moving.

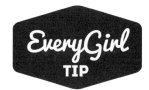

YOGI CAMERON ON HOT/COLD WATER

It comes down to hot versus cold. Clothes washed in hot water are cleaned better because the heat breaks up the dirt and allows the water to carry it away. Cold water shrinks the fibers in the cloth, not allowing the dirt to loosen up.

In our body it is the same. Cold causes us to contract, and hot to open up. An athlete who is 'warmed up' can perform better as their muscles are looser. Cold muscles, on the other hand, are tense and limited in their movement.

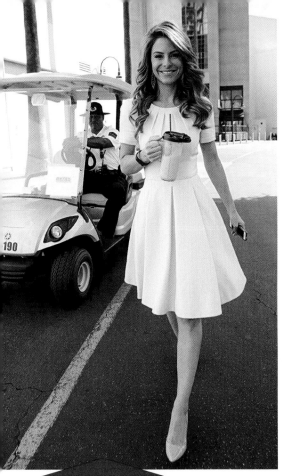

EveryGirl TIP

WALK FAST

When I was the ambassador for the Consumer Electronics Show, a large electronics convention, one of the things the CES staff remembered me for was how fast I walked in the two days I was there. When one of the guys remarked to Kev, "Is this how fast she always walks?" He replied, "Yep, how do you think she stays in such good shape?"

A lot of people like to think exercise has to come in large, sweat-soaked doses; believe me, I feel more accomplished when I do those kinds of workouts, too. But small, cumulative activity throughout the day is one of the main ways you burn calories, keep your metabolism stoked, and keep weight off—not to mention raise your energy levels, be more productive, and reduce stress.

One example is just walking. As I said, *Extra* has a golf cart to take Mario and me to any place on the set we need to go, but when time allows, I opt to walk instead. I'm always taking stairs in lieu of elevators and walking briskly when I do.

Trainer to the stars and good friend Harley Pasternak got me hooked on counting my daily steps, and wearing a wristband pedometer to keep track of how far I've walked each day. I've made it my goal to take ten thousand steps as I go about my day and find that I can maintain my current shape by doing that. Because I don't engage in routine daily or even weekly workouts, walking ten thousand steps is the perfect goal and substitute. And overall, I carry a sense of urgency in my workdays, purposely walking to and from desks and through corridors at a brisk pace, and I know it helps.

If you can find ways to squeeze in activity here and there, that's where the weight-loss battle is won. Yes, structured exercise can be important, too, but it's more important simply to be moving. On a conference call, stand up and pace. Watching your toddlers at the park? Stop sitting on the bench and walk laps around the perimeter. Meeting your girlfriends for coffee three times a week? Suggest taking a hike or going for a walk in the park on one of those days instead. At the airport, never use the moving sidewalks. At malls, forget the escalators and take the stairs. At work, walk quickly to the water cooler, bathroom, conference room, or your coworker's office. I look at it like every bit counts and every bit of extra work I put in throughout my day means I have to spend less time at the gym. I do realize that gyms are great and have tools specifically designed to properly tone you. But don't overlook ABM, even if you do go to a gym consistently and get yourself in shape. ABM will help keep the weight off. You'll also find yourself accomplishing a lot more in your day, and that's positive and empowering.

EVERYGIRL RULE 9
Make Fitness Fun

Growing up with a lot of boys around me—I have tons of male first cousins!—we played a lot of sports. If it wasn't wrestling, it was street hockey. If it wasn't street hockey, it was football. If it wasn't football, it was basketball. We were always moving—competing, playing, having fun.

As I grew older, I started to play basketball for the boys' team in a youth church league. One of my cousins, Chris, was the coach, and his then-girlfriend (now his wife), Julie, was a very good basketball player. So I asked her to start a girls' team with us, and she did! I played on that team and eventually played in high school. I wasn't all that good, but I was a hustler and a scrapper. And most important, I discovered something I really loved. I enjoy my workouts, but for me playing sports like basketball is way more fun. And because it's fun, I'm far more motivated to do it.

One of my favorite things to do is call a bunch of friends (both men and women) and invite them

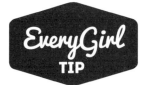

Every Girl TIP

MARIA'S FUN FITNESS WITH FRIENDS

Exercise activities I constantly do with friends that are healthier than going out to eat and drink and are THE best of bonding times:

Weekend hikes

ANY chance to play semi-organized team sports, whether it's flag football, pick-up volleyball, or hoop games

5K runs

Dance classes

Dog-walking dates

Workouts splitting the training fees

↓ My crew from *Extra* on my court. We go all out when we play!

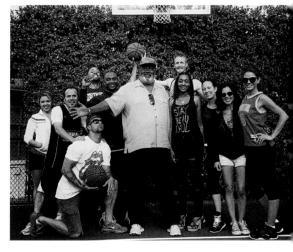

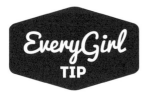

EveryGirl TIP

PICK UP AN ELECTRONIC WRISTBAND

Electronic wristbands that measure how many steps you take sell for under $100. Many even measure the calories you burn during the day. Not only are they a great tool for tracking your steps, but they serve as a constant reminder to keep moving.
I like wristbands best. I find pedometers that attach to your shoes fall off frequently. They are also inconvenient should you want to change shoes. I wear my FitBit bracelet all the time.

to a game of basketball and a barbecue. These afternoon parties often last well into the evening. We're having so much fun sweating, competing, and laughing with each other that we don't want it to end. It's a key lesson: Doing something physical that you *like* to do is motivating, and doing it with people you care about makes it even more so. *Dancing with the Stars* was another great example of

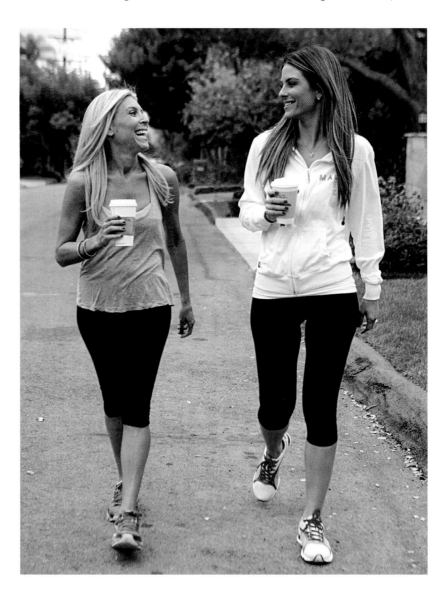

→ Instead of sitting for coffee, we walk with it. Well, Rachel has coffee; I have hot water!

getting fit by having fun. I made friends, discovered something new, overcame challenges, built confidence and got my body in the best shape it's ever been.

In part 3 of this book, I'm going to give you lots of ideas for workouts. However, no matter how effective the workout, if you're not enjoying it at least to some extent, you'll bail on it. Ask yourself what activity, exercise, or sport you love and then pursue it.

EVERYGIRL RULE 10
Make No Comparisons

Pam Anderson has the most amazing body. No wait, Gisele Bündchen has the most amazing body. Actually, Kim Kardashian has the most amazing body. Or is it Kristen Stewart? Natalie Portman, Beyoncé, Rihanna, J-Lo? I haven't a clue as to the answer, and guess what? No one else does, either. It's all subjective, which is why it's not worth comparing ourselves to them or anyone else. Those women all have different body types that are appealing. Kim will never have Gisele's body and Gisele will never have Kim's body. Neither is better, necessarily; they're just different. It's pointless in business and in life to compare yourself to others, and the same goes for body types and appearance. If you admire someone's body, whether it's a celebrity, a friend, or an acquaintance, feel free to study the techniques they're using, just as you are now studying mine. However, adopt those habits to get *your* best body, not someone else's body. Comparing yourself to others in unhealthy and obsessive ways, the way I've seen many girls do, can make you discouraged and depressed. How is that going to get you healthy and fit? It isn't. It's only going to waste time and energy—two things we need to conserve to be successful in any of our goals, including health and fitness.

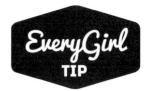

OPT TO WEAR FLATS AT WORK...
Or any other comfortable shoe when you can. Flats are still fashionable and yet easier to walk fast in. When I have to wear heels I maintain my urgency as best I can, but it's not as comfortable and not as safe. If you have to wear heels to work, maybe you can keep a pair of flats at your desk for the day-to-day hustle.

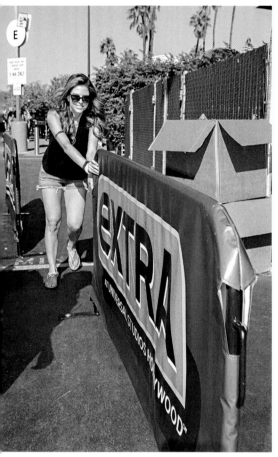

↑ I decided to pitch in and help the crew at *Extra* pack up so I could take them all for some rides at the Universal theme park. I take any chance I can get to be physical.

Do What Works for You!

As I said in the introduction, talk to different trainers, dietitians, or doctors and you'll hear different, and sometimes quite rigid, beliefs on the subjects of diet and fitness. However, everyone's body *and mind* respond differently to various techniques. What helps one person lose weight, get toned, or become healthy may not work for someone else. In addition, what motivates or inspires each individual can be very different.

When Kev had that bout of depression, his energy was very low, and as a result, he had cravings for those unhealthy quick-energy foods. As you might guess, he grew out of shape. But being the smart guy that he is, he knew that exercise would improve his mood and help him get fit at the same time. He did some research on workout machines and decided to buy a Bowflex. Trainer friends of mine made fun of him for getting one and told me what a waste of money it was and how little he'd be able to achieve with it. I initially jumped on the bandwagon. Surely the experts knew better. But what the experts didn't know was Kev. To him, there were lots of advantages. In addition to providing resistance training, which he had read was crucial for fitness, Kev liked the fact the Bowflex was space-saving as well as cheaper and more convenient than joining a gym. It was a machine he could use safely on his own, and we could also use it together. He bought it, he used it regularly, and he improved his fitness and his depression. Maybe hiring a trainer and joining a high-tech gym would have gotten him in better shape, but maybe the extra time needed to commute to the gym would have caused him to quit. Maybe the cost of a gym and a trainer would have done the same. Simply put, the Bowflex may not be right for some expert trainers, but it worked for Kev, and that was all that mattered. When it comes to fitness, whatever works for you, whatever you can afford, whatever you can live with, whatever you enjoy, whatever motivates you is what you should do.

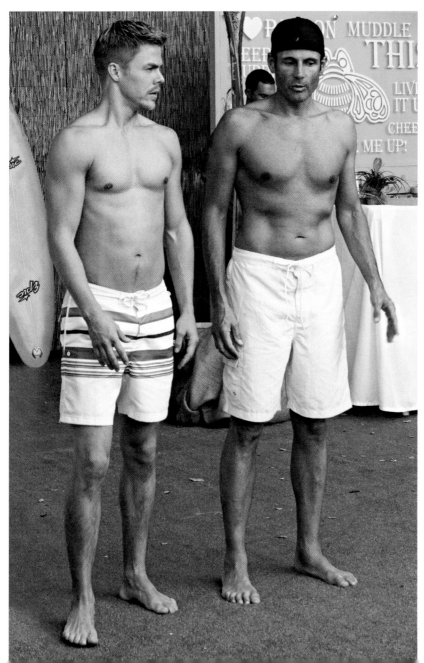

← Kev's body ranking right up there with Derek Hough, 20 years his junior, who's a pro dancer! Keven's got a great body, and he did it without trainers, using home workout equipment that "experts" claimed wouldn't work.

Q What keeps you inspired to exercise and watch what you eat? Do you use any mantras?

My biggest mantra is: Don't look at the scale; don't be a slave to that number. The number that you should be concerned with is seven, and that is to be active every single day of the week. I am, and just knowing that I am doing something daily that is an investment in myself and my future makes me feel better. Another one of my mottos: Just have fun. And if it's not fun, then make it fun. Working out isn't exactly the most fun thing we can do, but I wear bright colors to the gym, and I have a good playlist of songs to motivate me. One of the most motivating things is results. Once you start seeing results, that's so inspiring.

Q What is your philosophy on weight loss?

My philosophy is just do it now, and slowly. Have realistic expectations. TV shows like The Biggest Loser *have warped people's perception as to how long it should take you to become fitter. It shouldn't happen in a matter of weeks. For me it's been years, and thankfully it's been building and building and improving over time, and I'm still tweaking and working on my own things. It's really a lifestyle change, if anything. As they say, it's a complete rewiring of the brain.*

Q What is your philosophy on health?

The healthier I have become, the happier I have become. So, a healthier person is a happier person, and don't we all want to live happier lives?

Q What's your best advice for someone struggling to lose weight?

My best advice is just walk! Walking is underrated. Walk every day for at least thirty minutes a day, and that will help you. Walking will not hurt, everyone knows how to do it, it's free, you don't need any equipment, and you have no excuses.

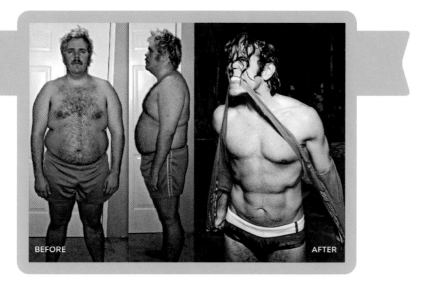

BEFORE

AFTER

What's one food people should think of subtracting and one food they should think of adding to their regular diet?

Subtracting from their diet: ice cream. Ice cream is just bad news all around. Adding: kale. Add it to your smoothies and protein shakes—it makes it so fibrous and dense it's almost like a meal replacement. And also, bake your kale and enjoy it as kale chips. Add a little seasoning, and it's so healthy and good for you.

What are your other favorite healthy snacks? What do you grab on the go?

I love fat-free Greek yogurt. You can't go wrong with that. You can get it at most delis or convenience stores. It's high in protein, low in fat and sugars. I love it.

What are a few of your favorite workouts?

I discovered a great new workout recently that's called Tabata, which is amazing for fat burning, and I am loving that.

How do you deal with guilt when you've eaten something not in line with your goals or missed a workout?

I don't have much guilt these days, because I work so hard at the gym, and I'm so consistent. So when I do cheat I'm like, "Okay, whatever," it will just slow my progress it's not going to derail it."

85

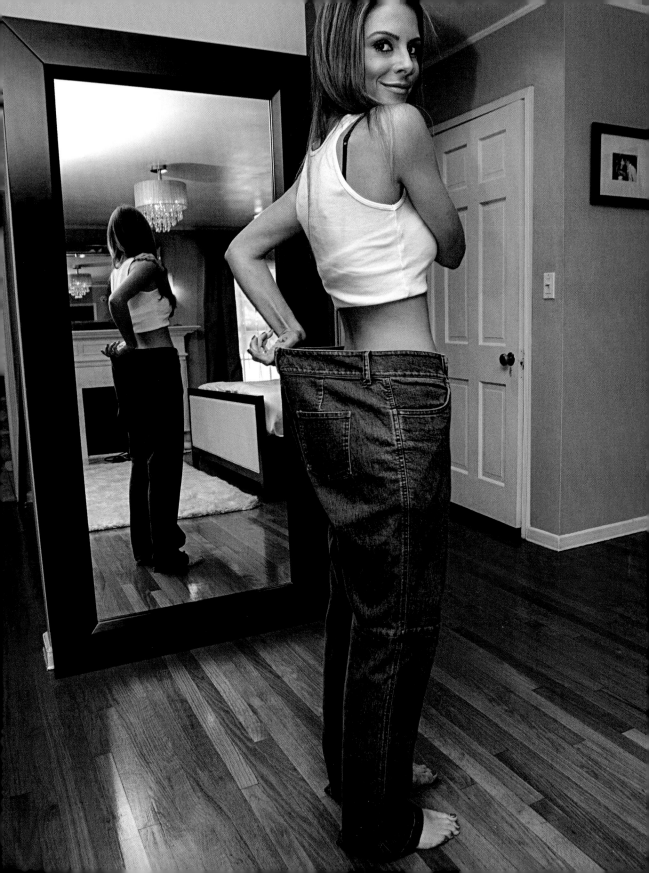

PART TWO

EveryGirl

DIET

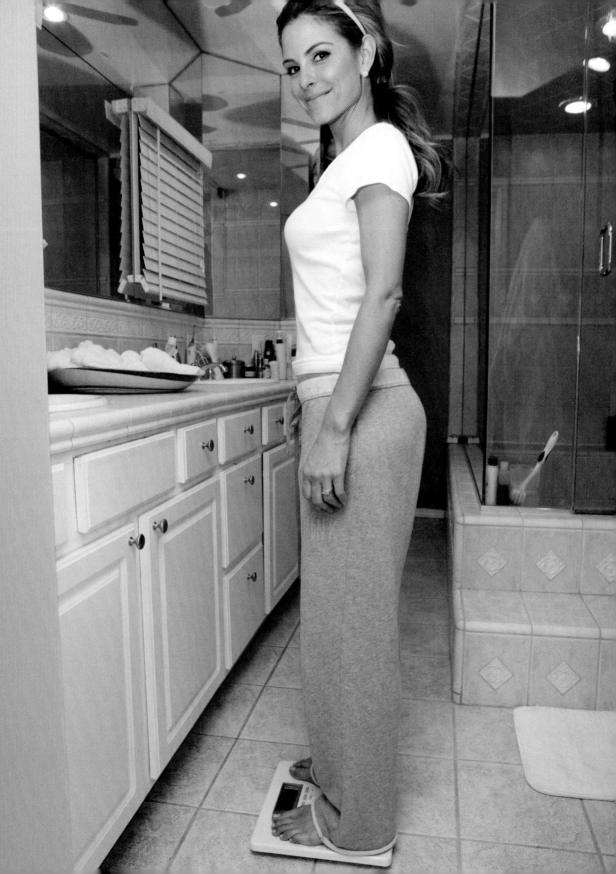

Chapter 5

My EveryGirl Weight-Loss Journey:

The thirteen steps that helped me drop forty pounds—and keep them off for good!

Baby had back!

In case you're wondering, those oversized jeans you see me wearing in the section opener are the actual pants I wore when I was heavier. I've kept them all these years as a reminder and an inspiration to always put my health first.

When people hear that I lost forty pounds years ago and haven't regained the weight, the first thing they say is, "How did you do it?"

Well, here are the no-time, no-money steps I followed—back when I had no time and no money! And honestly, though my circumstances have changed, if I gained the weight back today, these are the basic steps I'd repeat.

Phase One

These steps consist of two phases. Phase One is where you start. These steps are more basic and easier to follow; however, they're crucial to your attaining success in Phase Two and overall.

STEP 1
Set a Deadline

You can't just say, "I want to lose weight. . .someday." It's that kind of loose talk, without a fence or guideline, that discourages you from getting started and prevents you from succeeding. The way I did it was by tying it to an upcoming event in my life, which I'll explain soon. I never focused on a number and I didn't set out to lose a certain number of pounds per week or overall. I merely found a target date a year away and proclaimed to myself that I'd be in better shape by then.

My goal was to stop overeating and aim to be healthier, slowly dropping the weight. I knew I had the entire year to gradually make changes that would yield me the results I was looking for.

Tie It to an Upcoming Event in Your Life

Aiming for a deadline like this gives you necessary motivation. Maybe you want to get in shape for an upcoming class or family reunion or wedding—someone else's or your own. Maybe you're

THE EVERYGIRL'S GUIDE TO DIET AND FITNESS

STEPPING OUT OF YOUR COMFORT ZONE

There's nothing wrong with tying your weight-loss goal to an event such as a wedding or class reunion. But consider stepping out of your comfort zone. Whether doing pageants, or even Dancing with the Stars, *I stepped out of my comfort zone and tried something new and got positive results. A pageant or even a local dance competition (since* Dancing with the Stars, *they've popped up all over the place) might be a good step for you. Today, they have such competitions and exhibitions for people of all ages. These are amazing because you get to learn how to dance, which is fun, PLUS the actual training involved in dance will help you to lose weight and get fit. My body was never more toned than when I competed on* DWTS.

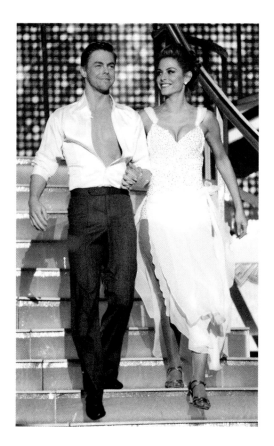

You don't want to be too focused on the competition, though. That will just stress you out and even set you up for failure. When I was involved with Dancing with the Stars, *I never talked about winning or even thought about it. Derek will tell you that, and he said that was one of the reasons he liked working with me. I was all about hanging in as long as I could because it was such an amazing experience. Whether it's a pageant, dance competition, or road race, mirror that attitude. You'll have more fun and not be stressed—and fun is what you deserve!*

going on vacation and want to look great on the beach. Maybe you want to run a marathon, which is amazing because your event involves exercise.

My event at the time was the Miss Massachusetts USA pageant. I knew the show had a swimsuit portion, and if I was going to be in a bathing suit in front of thousands of people, I wanted to be in the best possible shape. I decided to enter the competition in January 1999—the pageant was in November—leaving me eleven months to get bathing-suit ready. There was a significant entrance fee, too. I knew that if I didn't get in shape, I wouldn't be able to compete and would be wasting money. Financial stakes motivated me even more.

Be Patient

Determine that moment in the future when you wish to have the weight off, but remember: It's a marathon, not a sprint. The longer it takes to lose the weight, the easier it is to do and the more likely you are to keep it off. It's reasonable and doable to lose a pound a week. That may not sound like a lot, but that's twenty-five pounds in six months. If you don't lose the desired amount of weight by your deadline it's okay. The deadline is just there to get you started and provide some structure for your journey.

Keep It to Yourself

When I first applied these steps, I didn't tell anyone, and neither should you. I didn't know whether I would succeed, and by telling others I felt as though I was just putting even more pressure on myself. Weight loss is tough enough to achieve—why make it any harder? Five months into my weight-loss journey, my mom asked me whether I was losing weight, but other than that no one had any idea, and it allowed me to work at my own pace.

STEP 2
Weigh Yourself

Now that you've established your event and deadline date, step on the scale and weigh yourself. This will give you a starting weight you can gauge your success by later. Once you've written down your start weight PUT THE SCALE AWAY. I don't want you to step on it until later in these steps. Hopping on the scale on a daily or even weekly basis will set you up for disappointment, discouragement, and failure. That's why I didn't do it, and you shouldn't, either.

STEP 3
Buy a Journal

Now that you've set your weight loss goal, congratulations! Next, I want you to buy some kind of diary to serve as your weight-loss journal. Any spiral notebook will do. That's all I used. But maybe you can spring for a leather-bound one, which can cost you as little as ten dollars. The professional look and feel may motivate you even more to fill it out every day. Plus, it'll last longer, which is cool because for a food journal to be effective, you may need to refer back to it frequently.

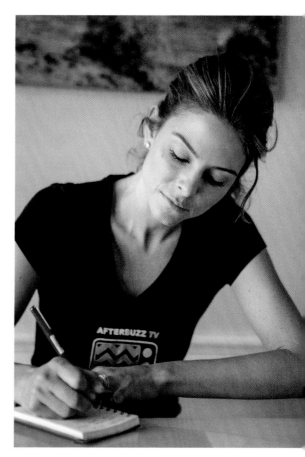

STEP 4
Write Down Everything You Eat in a Week

Before you begin to change your diet, spend a week recording everything you eat—and I mean *everything*. Before I made any changes to my

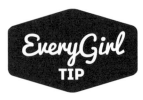

EveryGirl TIP

PACK IT TO GO

I have Tupperware and Ziploc bags in all shapes and sizes. I load them up every day with my healthy snacks, such as sliced apples, carrots, and celery, or nuts and berries. If healthy food is there and easy, I'll grab it.

diet, I journaled everything I ate each day for a week, including little things like gum or breath mints. If you have a piece of candy from your coworker's desk, snag a few spoonfuls of your boyfriend's ice cream, or finish the few bits of grilled cheese your kid left on her plate, write it down! It all adds up, and you just don't realize how much you're eating until you actually see it all on paper in front of you. I, for one, was stunned. Seeing it all in black and white was an eye-opener and a breakthrough for me. Remember what I said about having the courage to take responsibility for your own actions and how many of us are in denial and blame outside forces when it comes to personal problems? I was in such denial about my eating. I never thought I ate much more than any other girl. I used to blame my body type for the extra forty pounds I was carrying around. However, when I saw it all on paper, there was no denying that I was simply eating too much food and too much of the wrong kind of food. After journaling, I was able to fully accept that being unhealthy was my fault—something I'd created and something only I could fix.

Carry your journal with you and fill it out whenever you eat anything. Don't wait until the end of the day when you might (conveniently) forget. When you write down what you ate, also write down when you ate it. It may help you spot patterns. This all may seem like a big pain, but studies show that women who keep a food journal lose six pounds more than women who don't.

STEP 5
Review and Assess What You Ate

At the end of the week, after the shock of seeing what you've been eating wears off, take a closer look at your diet. What are your problem areas? Are you eating too much sugar? Too much

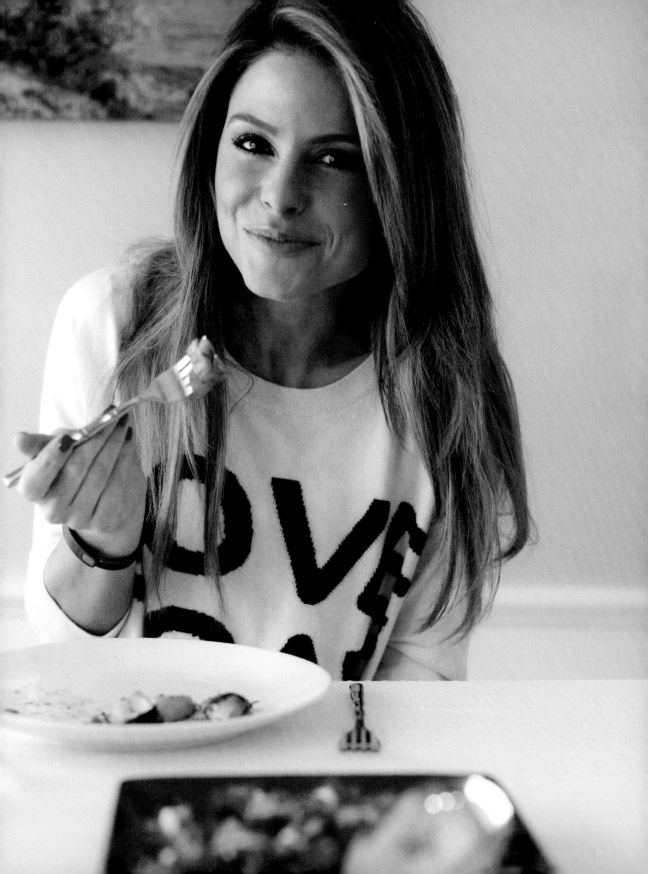

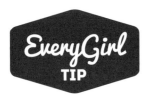

EveryGirl TIP

**TRY THE
TEN PERCENT RULE**

Try cutting back on food portions at a rate of 10 percent a week. It's a small enough number to adhere to easily, but big enough to help you achieve big results in the long term.

chocolate? Too much bread? Are you drinking too much alcohol? Are you eating late at night? I didn't have to be a dietitian to know that my biggest problem was carbs. I was eating tons of them. Cutting carbs, therefore, became my focus.

STEP 6
Cut Back Slowly

Now that you know what you're eating, it's time to deal with some of those trouble areas. As I said, mine was carbs—lots of pasta and lots of breads. I especially ate a ton of pizza. In Boston, between chains like Pizza Regina and Papa Gino's and the local mom-and-

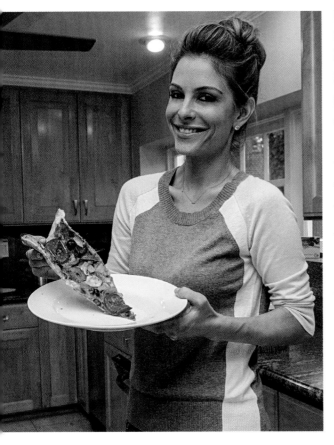

pop places, you are surrounded by the most amazing pizza in the entire world. I know this might be hard for you to believe, but back then I could eat seven slices of pizza in one sitting. I decided to make this one of the first things to cut back on.

So instead of seven slices of pizza, I would eat six. I know that doesn't seem like much of a cutback, but remember, we're not doing a 180. We're taking small steps. And even with this tiny adjustment, it was still hard to say no. But soon enough, it became less painful, and then I cut down to five slices.

When I finally made it down to three slices, I started to incorporate a salad. It was a healthier way to feel full and made it even easier to keep cutting back.

Most serious dieters would look at my chart and say, "You're overweight, Maria, because you eat a ton of pizza, so you need to cut that out." Never have pizza again? That would be so painful and discouraging! And again, how would feeling like that help me at a time when I needed to be positive and strong for the journey ahead?

You may keep cutting back and then permanently eliminate certain foods altogether from your diet. In my case this didn't happen with pizza, but it did with other unhealthy foods.

When I was learning to cut back, but I really wanted a little more food, I found tricks to help keep me on track. Here are a few of the things I did, and still do, to avoid overeating:

GET UP AND TAKE A WALK
During a meal, a walk even to the bathroom will create enough time for your brain to catch up to your stomach and realize it's full.

DRINK YOUR TRUSTED HOT WATER
At that point of eating when you know you should stop, drink some hot water or hot water with lemon. It will help fill you up and, again, buy your brain the time it needs.

SLEEP THE HUNGER OFF
Go to sleep, even if it's early. You'll wake up feeling no worse for wear.

MUNCH ON SOMETHING BETTER, LIKE APPLES
Instead of reaching for that third or fourth slice of pizza, grab an apple or a handful of carrots instead.

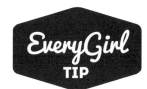

FILL UP ON VEGGIES!
If you need more food at a meal, then serve yourself an extra helping of vegetables. They have the fewest calories of any food and therefore will do the least dietary damage. Plus the fiber they contain fills you up, so you can't really overeat them.

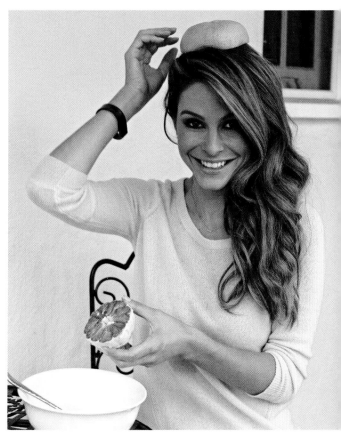

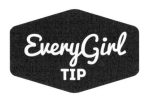

**THE
COMPANY LINE**

As I said, I never used the word *diet* in this process. I also never told anyone else I was attempting to lose weight—not even Keven. If I failed, I wanted to fail on my own, not in front of an audience. Should anyone notice that you are cutting back and inquire what you are up to, the company line, the line you'll have deeply embedded in your brain, is that you are just trying to make a few better choices in your eating habits. And by the way, you should be telling yourself that line, too. It's true and, again, it puts less pressure on you.

Phase Two

When you notice your clothes are fitting looser, congratulations. It's time to move on to Phase Two. Now, the transition to Phase Two could come at the six-month mark, or it could come sooner, or even later. It's simply that moment when you know what you've been doing is working. For me, there's no better cue than how my clothes fit.

Of course, you can disregard the first six steps, or even rush through them, and jump to Phase Two before you see any results. This book is all about you finding what works best for you. Remember, as evidenced from my experience, the longer you take to lose weight, the longer it will stay off. What I unknowingly did (and hope you will too), was spend five months learning how to slowly make better decisions. It wasn't every minute of every day. I wasn't counting calories or working out religiously. I was engaging in a gradual process that cumulatively, over time, gave way to permanent healthy habits that helped me maintain my weight loss. I remember going out to eat with Keven and hearing him say, "Honey just get a salad with your burger instead of the fries." I would look at him as if he was crazy and I'd actually get mad. Before I started losing weight, that was impossible to my brain. But when I focused on making these small changes, it all got easier. You essentially need to, and can, retrain your mind and appetite, but that takes time. The first six steps will begin that process, and the following steps in Phase Two will take you to the finish line.

STEP 7
Weigh Yourself Again

By May, five months into my process, my mom noticed I was losing weight. I was caught off guard by her comment, but I did notice my clothes were getting a bit baggy. Could it be that after all these years

I was finally losing weight? Remember, I weighed only myself once when I began the steps and then I quickly put the scale away. The only way to tell whether I was truly losing weight, and to what degree, was by steeping on the scale, so I pulled it out of my closet and hopped on. I discovered I had lost 20 pounds! It was the most overwhelming feeling of exhilaration and accomplishment. I remember, at my peak weight, grabbing fat on the side of my thigh and thinking, "How will this ever go away?" I really didn't think it was possible.

I succeeded because the first six steps in my plan were so simple. All I really did was cut back slowly and make a few healthy substitutions. And because I didn't tell anyone or incessantly hop on the scale, there was virtually no pressure. I quietly tricked my body into being sated by smaller quantities in the process.

Seeing I had lost 20 pounds recharged my motivation; I felt stronger, more committed and ready to take things to the next level.

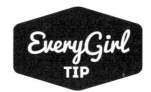

LIMIT STEPPING ON THE SCALE

During Phase Two You can step on the scale now and then, but do so only periodically. The scale is a decent barometer but it still doesn't measure health, and obsessing over the number on the scale can become an unhealthy obsession.

Don't Let Weight-Loss Plateaus Discourage You

Dieters often experience weight-loss plateaus, where they'll lose weight consistently, and then suddenly stop, for an extended period of time. This could happen to you, especially if your goal is to lose a significant amount of weight. But if you limit your visits to the scale you are less likely to notice them and less likely to get discouraged. And this is why I recommend taking your time with weight loss, so you can ride through the plateaus. And if you stick with the plan (and stay off the scale), in time, you will.

STEP 8
Go Back to Journaling

From this point on, it's not merely about cutting back; it's about smarter choices. Any time you can choose something healthier in your days, do it. If you recall in Step 4, I had you write down

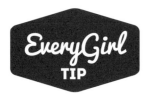

LIMIT THE BAD CARBS

The carb items I limited when I fine-tuned my diet were the bad ones as seen in refined grains, sweets, and breads. There are good carbs found in fruits, vegetables, legumes, and whole grains; but those were not the ones I limited.

Later in the book is a full breakdown and explanation of good carbs and bad carbs.

everything you ate for the first week. The reason I didn't do any more journaling in Phase One was because it was too cumbersome and time consuming. Those factors would only present more obstacles to a task that seemed impossible to achieve. After I lost the first 20 pounds, I was a girl on a mission and more than up for the task of journaling my food daily—as you will, no doubt, be.

Journaling everything I ate from that point until my pageant was essential because it kept me even more responsible for what was going into my body. I needed to see in black and white what I was choosing to eat every day and what physical activity I was doing. It served as a daily reminder to keep me more focused than ever. As I look back at my old logs, there were days I was really on target, eating healthily and getting a good workout in. Other days, I noted I was depressed and didn't work out. Another I noted that I did so well in my workout that I was ready to increase my exercises the following week. I still wasn't depriving myself of the things I loved most. One day I had a small steak and cheese sub and ice cream, but I had only a cup of ice cream. I was still enjoying things, but keeping the portions manageable. This will help you down the line with maintenance and having checks and balances. I certainly have days when I overindulge, but the next day I know I need to balance it out and eat cleaner. These are the lessons and habits that get ingrained in you when you take it slowly

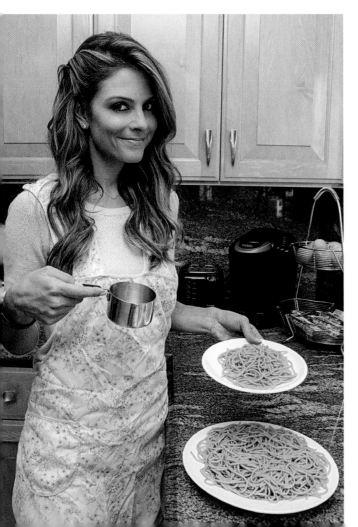

← I was shocked when I actually started measuring my pasta! We are so used to bigger portions! Fashion note: I'm wearing my late yiayia's apron. Miss her.

and focus on making better decisions, not what the scale says. I also used Weight Watchers meals from time to time. They were an easy addition to my diet because I could easily track my calories and macronutrients (protein, carbohydrates, fat). Also, they were convenient when I came home hungry and tired and didn't want to cook! And no, I wasn't paid by WeightWatchers to say that. There are lots of low-calorie meals you may want to have in the freezer for the same reason. The only way I even recall using WeightWatchers meals is because I wrote them in my journal. I still journal from time to time, whether it's for a shoot or just tying to clean up my diet a bit.

Your Phase Two Journal

This journal will need to be more detailed than it was in Phase One. I want you to write down not only what you are consuming, but also the approximate nutritional information, which may include calories and grams of protein, carbohydrates, and fat. Additionally, write about any exercise or physical activity you incorporate into your day. Note that you're recording protein intake because your muscles will need it. We'll discuss why later in the book. Below is a sample of what my phase two journal looked like. I added the totals at the bottom and wrote down any exercise activity below that.

MONDAY	JUNE 10			
	PROTEIN	CARBS	FAT	CALORIES
BREAKFAST Cereal w/skim	14	30	0	190

HERE'S WHAT I AIMED FOR:

CALORIES: around 1,500 calories

PROTEIN: 50-100 grams

FAT: less than 60 grams

CARBS: less than 200 grams

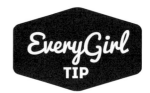

THE FITNESS PAL APP

The Fitness Pal app allows you to easily maintain a food diary by scanning the bar codes on any food items purchased at a grocery store. It instantly uploads nutrition facts and serving size into your diary and allows you to track your daily calorie count. You can input exercise workouts, too, to track calorie burning.

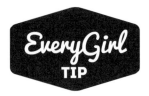

The Formula to Determine Daily Calories

Don't let the math problem below scare you, the formula for healthy and successful weight loss isn't complicated, and it's one you can adjust once you've reached your goal weight.

YOU MAY NOT BE ABLE TO SHRINK YOUR STOMACH BUT YOU CAN SHRINK YOUR APPETITE

Many people believe that if they eat less over a long period of time they can shrink their stomachs and therefore the need for more food. Experts contend there is no such thing as shrinking your stomach by eating less. The stomach expands when it takes in food, then returns to its same size when food passes. However, when you do eat less, something IS proven to shrink: your appetite. And with a smaller appetite, you're bound to eat less anyhow.

_____

x 10

_____ =

YOUR WEIGHT

YOUR RESTING METABOLIC RATE
(how many calories your body needs to function on a daily basis without any movement at all)

X _____

_____ =

ACTIVITY FACTOR (below)

ESTIMATED CALORIC NEEDS
(the number of calories needed to maintain your weight)

ACTIVITY FACTOR

1.3	1.5	1.6	1.9
SEDENTARY	LIGHT	MODERATE	VERY ACTIVE
throughout the day (vegging in front of the TV)	(desk job)	(if you have an active job like waiting tables or exercise daily)	(if you're an athlete or exercise for multiple hours each day)

If you weigh 130 pounds and have a desk job, the formula for your estimated caloric needs would look like this:

130 x 10 = 1,300 calories x 1.5 = 1,950

If you want to lose weight, you would then subtract 300–500 calories a day, so if you weigh 130 pounds, you would need to eat between 1,450 and 1,650 calories a day.

The great thing about this formula is that once you achieve your goal weight, you can use it to calculate how many calories you need to maintain that weight. In that case, simply redo the formula with your new weight and don't subtract those 300–500 calories.

STEP 9
Fine-Tune Your Diet

I learned in Phase One that my problem area was carbs such as refined grains, breads, pasta, and pizza, and I cut back slowly on them. In Phase Two, however, I strove to cut down to only one of those carb items per day. I could choose to eat it for breakfast, lunch, or dinner. If pasta was on the menu for dinner, then that was my one carb for the day. I wouldn't just rest on that, though. I was also mindful of portion control. In the case of pasta, for example, I would measure out one cup. Since I made the decision to try to keep my caloric intake to under 1,500 per day, I was also reading more and more labels and doing more research on nutritional values in general.

You, too, may want to consume only one major carb item per day, of the ones containing refined grains as in pizza, pasta, and breads, and to eat under 1,500 calories per day in total. Later in the book, I go deeper into explaining the difference between the bad carbs and the good ones as well as other beneficial nutritional facts.

My One Serving of Carbs a Day
When I eventually scaled back my diet to one carb a day—good or bad carb—these were some of my options. (I know it seems impossible now, but trust me, it gets easier. I still aim for this today!)

100% WHOLE-GRAIN BREAD: Bread goes with just about everything, so it's important to remember that a serving is one slice.

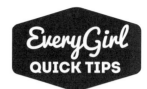

EveryGirl QUICK TIPS

AVOID JUNK AND PROCESSED FOODS
Eat real, whole foods as much as possible.

KEEP YOUR HOME FREE OF JUNK AND FATTY FOODS
Out of sight, out of mind.

AVOID EATING AFTER 7PM
Drink water, find something to keep busy or hit the sack and sleep it off. If you must, have an apple, celery or carrots.

COOK YOUR OWN MEALS
This gives you ultimate control over ingredients and calories.

PACK A LUNCH TO WORK
Lends further control and helps avoid temptation. You can eat at your desk and free up your lunch hour to take a walk or even get a workout in.

LIMIT SOCIAL LUNCHES OR DINNERS
Its just more temptation and pressure. Try to create social occasions that don't revolve around food until you know you can handle it.

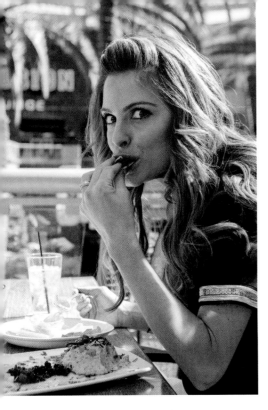

CEREAL: These days I'm a fan of Kashi GoLean and General Mills Fiber One. They are low in sugar and calories and high in fiber.

Special K and Cheerios are okay backups; that's what I ate back then. I cut anything with more than five grams of sugar per serving and *always* measured out one cup—it's so easy to abuse portion sizes with cereal.

PASTA: I would eat one cup of quinoa or brown rice pastas. Omit white-flour pasta, if possible, and make sure not to overeat.

PITA BREAD: Small whole-wheat pitas—I would eat one full one.

PIZZA: One slice loaded with vegetables is okay. Avoid eating the end crust to cut carbs, if possible.

↑ Having hummus at Karl Strauss at work. I love it and try to eat it with veggie sticks when I can instead of pita.

If You Like Dessert, Have It

Dessert is not forbidden. I didn't cut it out when I was losing weight, and I still enjoy it. In the next chapter, I'm going to discuss a simple way to work splurges into your weight-loss plan, but for now, know that a reasonable portion of dessert can definitely fit into your diet. However, that doesn't mean you have to have the most decadent dessert—and truthfully, you'll find that as you get used to eating better, heavy desserts with lots of sugar will leave you feeling so blah, you won't crave them as much. Here are a few tips for keeping dessert in your life.

➔ **Try low-fat options, including lower-fat frozen yogurts.** Or just have Greek yogurt. I recommend it, not just because I'm a proud Greek but also because it's high in protein. Protein builds muscle, fills you up, and keeps your metabolism humming. It's rich and thick and not as tangy as other yogurt—it's like eating ice

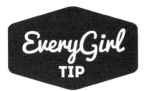

TIP

PICK UP A MAGIC BULLET BLENDER

I use mine constantly to blend healthy shakes and dressings. Fast to use, space saving, and easy to clean—they are a convenient kitchen and weight-loss companion.

THE EVERYGIRL'S GUIDE TO DIET AND FITNESS

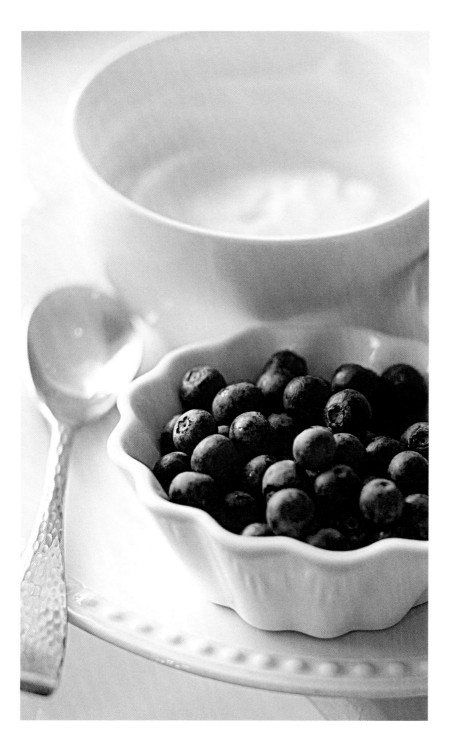

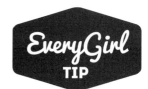

MAKE YOUR
OWN SALAD DRESSING

I love mixing lemon, olive oil, salt, pepper, and oregano in my Magic Bullet blender. I also love mixing vinegar, oil, basil, oregano, and rosemary. Homemade salad dressings are fresh, low calorie, and delicious!

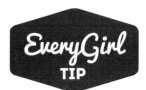

BEWARE
REFINED SUGAR

"Researchers now know that nutrition and cognition are closely linked-what's more important than brain health? Someday sugar will be classified as a drug-it's that addictive and that damaging. Sugar rehab – you heard it here first."

Michele Promaulayko
editor in chief,
Women's Health

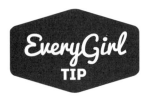

Every Girl TIP

FREEZE YOUR FRUIT
Try freezing bananas, berries, mangos, etc. It takes longer to eat frozen fruit, and feels more like a treat.

cream. Serve plain Greek yogurt with a little honey or some fresh fruit instead of the flavored yogurt, which has a lot of sugar.

Low-fat desserts are great for Phase Two, but once you've reached your goal weight and achieved a new and healthier relationship with food, you can start incorporating some of your full-fat favorites back into your diet.

➜ **Share Your Dessert.** Have only one or two bites—you'll be surprised how much a little bit satisfies you. This is a great strategy when you're out to dinner with friends—order one dessert for the table and let everyone share. You'll limit your intake of sugar, and your friends will be impressed by your generosity!

➜ **Pair a small portion of the treat with fruit.** For instance, have a thin slice of cake and top it with a cup of berries. Or serve sliced peaches with a half cup of ice cream. Chocolate and strawberries are divine.

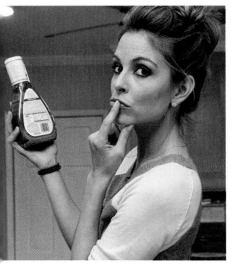

LEARN TO READ FOOD LABELS

Don't fall for claims on the front of the label, such as "all-natural" or "low-fat." "Low-fat" can mean high in sugar. You want to get in the habit of looking at the back of the package. Don't just check calories, either. Look at serving size. You may think you're buying a small package that serves one person, but the label may say there are three servings in that package. That means, if you scarfed that package down in a single go, you'd be eating three times the calories. Also look at the amount of sugar a food has and try to keep it as low as possible. Check fiber, too, and pick those foods that have plenty of it. Finally, read the small print: the ingredients list. The rule I use: The foods with the lowest number of ingredients are best, and the more words I don't recognize in the ingredients list, the worse the food probably is for me. Avoid foods with high-fructose corn syrup and trans fats especially.

→ **Read labels and limit servings.** There's nothing wrong with sating your sweet tooth, but be sure to read labels and know exactly what constitutes a serving size. Chips Ahoy! has a serving size of two cookies, with 120 calories and 5 grams of fat. When I was losing weight I made sure to stick to two cookies and track them in my food journal.

Get a High from Saying No

You've had whatever meal or treat you've put in your mouth a million times. You know how it tastes, and that high you experience from the taste—both of which last only a few minutes or even seconds. What you want instead is a new high: the high you'll get from being able to finally wear that fitted dress. That new high lasts a whole lot longer. Ultimately, try to get used to getting more of a high from saying "No, thank you" rather than "f–it I, give in." It works, and after a few times, it gets easier.

STEP 10
Start Exercising

I specifically didn't mention exercising in Phase One because I didn't exercise when I first started. I felt that the added pressure of exercise in the beginning of my weight loss journey was too overwhelming and could derail me from the slow and steady progress I was aiming for. Once I experienced the triumph of losing twenty pounds, I started working out three to four days a week. As usual, I started slowly. I didn't have enough stamina to do too much anyhow. You may not either—especially if exercise is new to you. I built up my exercise stamina, and over time, working out helped build more confidence and resolve. This is when I got a trainer involved, and in one session she outlined a plan I used to lose the last twenty pounds. It's featured in chapter 9 and in the workout section. You can use the plan like I did or any of the others you prefer in that section.

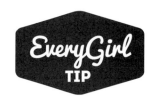

MAKE SUNDAY YOUR PREP DAY

On Sunday nights, I would prepare meals and snacks for the upcoming workweek. I would make a big batch of lima beans or lentils and keep it in the fridge. I also cut up fruits and veggies and placed them in Tupperware containers and Ziploc bags. If fruits and veggies aren't ready to eat, I get lazy and am less likely to consume them. The food in the fridge can be for a moment when you need a healthy snack, a meal, or something to take to work for lunch. It's definitely a little time consuming, but it puts YOU in control of your eating. I did this while working three jobs, so I know you can do it, too!

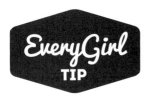

LEMON LAWS

Lemons, like grapefruit, are believed to produce an alkalizing effect in the body.

The alkaline diet, a diet that emphasizes eating foods with acid-neutralizing, or alkalizing properties, such as fruits, vegetables, nuts, and legumes, is thought to return balance to the acidity levels in our bodies. Often disturbed by acid producing foods like meat, grains and dairy.

While I don't do the alkaline diet per se, I've come to realize that much of what I eat really centers around the same principles of restoring balance, especially when it comes to eating lots of citrus fruits like lemon and grapefruit—which are acidic, but produce an alkaline effect in the body.

This may explain why, after a recent few unhealthy weeks of eating, I didn't gain much weight. I truly believe it was due to the half a lemon I added to my hot water throughout the day..

STEP 11
Drink Lots of Water

I used to cut lemon wedges and insert them into filled water jugs for added flavor. Little did I know that lemons are believed to help burn calories (more details on that in a bit). I would fill up on water with lemons all day, which greatly helped to suppress my appetite. You also can try hot water with lemon or plain hot water.

Eat Your Calories—Don't Drink Them!

A lot of drinks contain sugar and empty calories. Soda is the most obvious one, but also know that sports drinks, bottled ice tea, and flavored coffee drinks are usually packed with sugar. You can opt for artificially sweetened diet versions, but they aren't the healthiest alternatives. If you must have a diet soda, limit it to once a day. Studies have linked heavy diet soda consumption to weight gain. A Purdue University study found artificial sweeteners, like the ones used in diet sodas, disrupt the body's natural ability to regulate calorie intake based on the sweetness of foods. Simply put, sugar makes you crave sugar, and since your body can't tell the difference between natural and artificial sweeteners, fake sugar makes you crave sugar. Including artificially sweetened drinks in your diet may cause you to eat more. The calories in these drinks isn't the only problem. When you drink your calories, they aren't as satisfying, studies show. And that's proven true for me.

There may be a time when you want to have a cocktail, though. You can, but be careful.

Alcoholic Beverages

Alcohol by itself has calories, and when you mix it with fruit juice or other mixers that contain sugar, it only adds more. The added sugars in flavored martinis, piña coladas, margaritas, wine, and

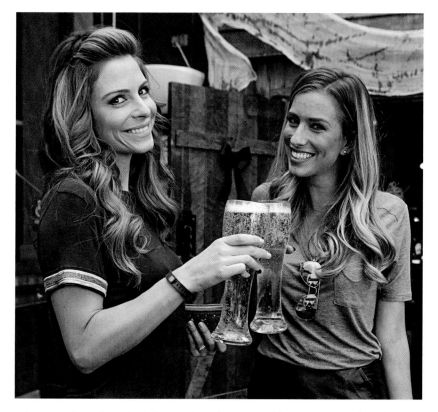

← I like light beer. Here with Renee Bargh, our *Extra* weekend show host on her b-day.

wine coolers just heighten the damage. Plus, getting drunk usually leads to other unhealthy habits such as overeating and late-night food bingeing. Hangovers also leave you craving and consuming unhealthy, greasy foods to soak up the alcohol.

Vodka is the one form of alcohol that's significantly lower in carbs. I recommend a quality vodka mixed with water or soda water with limes or lemons. At the end of the day, it's still unnecessary calories. However, this is a lighter, cleaner drink that has real fruit plus the hydrating factor of the water. (Alcohol dehydrates you, which is part of what leads to hangovers.) If you're really on your game, you'll drink a glass of water after every drink, further hydrating you while slowing down your alcohol consumption in the process.

When I was losing weight I didn't drink much at all. Today, I still don't drink all that often, but when I do I stick with a light beer or a glass of red wine. I recommend you limit alcohol consumption as much as possible in these 13 steps.

STEP 12
Get a Really Good Burn from Foods

There are actually foods out there that seem to be directly related to weight loss. One of them is grapefruit; in a study, researchers discovered that dieters who ate half a grapefruit before their meals lost more weight than those who didn't. So, when I fine-tuned my diet in Phases 2, I made grapefruit the first thing I ate each morning. (But don't worry, I'm not telling you that's all you should eat. I also had cereal and all kinds of different egg-white omelets..) And more studies have revealed other foods that help enhance weight loss in other ways. Keep in mind, this isn't a license to gorge. Eat these items in moderation. Back then I added hot peppers and spices to sandwiches, salads and anything I could, and I still do to this day.

HOT PEPPERS: Capsaicin, the compound that gives chili peppers their punch, heats up your body, which increases your metabolism so that you burn more calories. Enjoy them raw, cooked, dried, or even powdered. They're a great way to boost the flavor of other foods.

LEAN MEATS: Protein has a high thermogenic, or "heat-producing," effect in your body. That's because your body has to work harder to digest it, and it burns calories doing so!

ASPARAGUS: Asparagus is a natural diuretic. It flushes fluids and minimizes water-weight gain—especially after eating salty foods.

WHOLE GRAINS: Your body burns more calories breaking down whole foods that are rich in fiber rather than processed foods. Steel-cut oatmeal and brown rice are great examples.

LENTILS: My dad eats them every other day. One cup has more than a third of your daily iron needs. Many people, especially young women, are iron-deficient. That slows your metabolism, which can lead to weight gain. Lentils are a great diet addition to curb this. Lentils are also high in fiber, which takes longer to digest and keeps you feeling full, which further aids weight loss.

GREEN TEA: Epigallocatechin gallate, or EGCG, is a compound in green tea that temporarily speeds metabolism. Studies have shown that drinking green tea helps people lose weight.

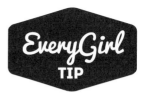

WHEN TO STOP

Our goal is to develop a new long-term diet and fitness lifestyle, but there's also a time to ease up. When you feel better and are happy with your results, slowly add back some of your favorite foods in moderation. Just maintain portion control.

STEP 13
Rejoice and Reward!

And ta-da! By the time the pageant came around I had lost forty pounds! It took me about a year, but I did it and had tons more energy as a result. Because my clothes no longer fit, I had to buy a new wardrobe. Even though it was a practical thing, it was a great reward and something I recommend you do, too. I was broke at the time, but I was still able to piece together an inexpensive wardrobe. If you can't buy all-new clothes, do something else to reward yourself for your amazing efforts. Try not to reward yourself with food, though. A reward shouldn't open the door to returning to old eating habits.

Be Careful Not to Overdo It

I ended up losing five pounds more than I needed to. And that's not particularly healthy, either. Be mindful of losing too much weight.

These days I don't know what my daily calorie consumption is, but I still try to limit myself to one bad carb a day, and of course, smaller portions.

The rest of this book will show you how you can enhance all of the skills you've learned in Phase Two, and how you can maintain your success.

Q What's your fitness mantra?

Today is a new day. Yesterday doesn't matter anymore.

Q What's your philosophy on weight loss?

It's all about finding balance in your body physically, but also mentally. It's also about being very in tune with which foods your body does well with and the foods that make you feel bad and cause you problems. It is never about deprivation. It's never about eating fat-free or even low-fat foods. I'm a big believer in healthy fats.

Q How do you stay motivated to exercise and eat healthy?

My best motivator for keeping active changes from one day to the next. Sometimes waking up sluggish or in a head space I don't want to be in is all I need to get moving. Most important is carving out a routine for yourself, so you can devote a certain amount of time to exercise on a very regular basis. It's harder to make excuses and talk yourself out of it if it is regularly built into your day.

Q What is your advice for someone struggling to lose weight?

Drink a lot of water (sometimes hunger pains are actually dehydration). Cut out sugar and processed foods. It will be a shock to your system, in a good way. I try to keep my glycemic index down, so I really avoid sugar as much as possible, including juices.

Q Describe your typical diet.

I personally do well with red meat, eggs, leafy greens, fruits, nuts, and food high in iron. I eat a lot of protein. I've really been focusing lately on avoiding processed foods. I have not eliminated dairy altogether (I love it and I don't want to deprive myself of it), but I have cut way down. I have switched from low-fat milk to whole milk because it is

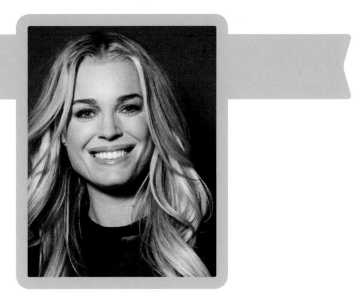

*less processed, and I add it only to my scrambled eggs in the morning.
I drink my coffee black. It took some getting used to, but now I like it.*

Q What's your favorite healthy snack?

*When I have a busy day and I need a snack I can grab on the go,
I go for apples and almonds. My favorite are Fuji apples. Refrigerated.
Yum. The fiber in the skin of apples is really good for your digestion and
helps keep your tummy flat.*

Q What is your fitness routine like?

*My goal is to break a sweat every day. It doesn't always happen;
usually I end up working out four days a week. I have most of my
energy in the morning, so I work out right after I drop my kids off at
school. I try to switch it up as much as possible: yoga, hiking, swimming,
Pilates, elliptical machine. Sometimes a good, long bike ride.*

Q How do you deal with the guilt of eating something you "shouldn't" or skipping a workout?

*I rarely feel guilty about treating myself. I like to have desserts and ice
cream with my kids. But if I've really gone for it, I get over it the next day
by waking up and knowing that it was worth it and that today is a new
day. Yesterday doesn't matter anymore. And I get moving.*

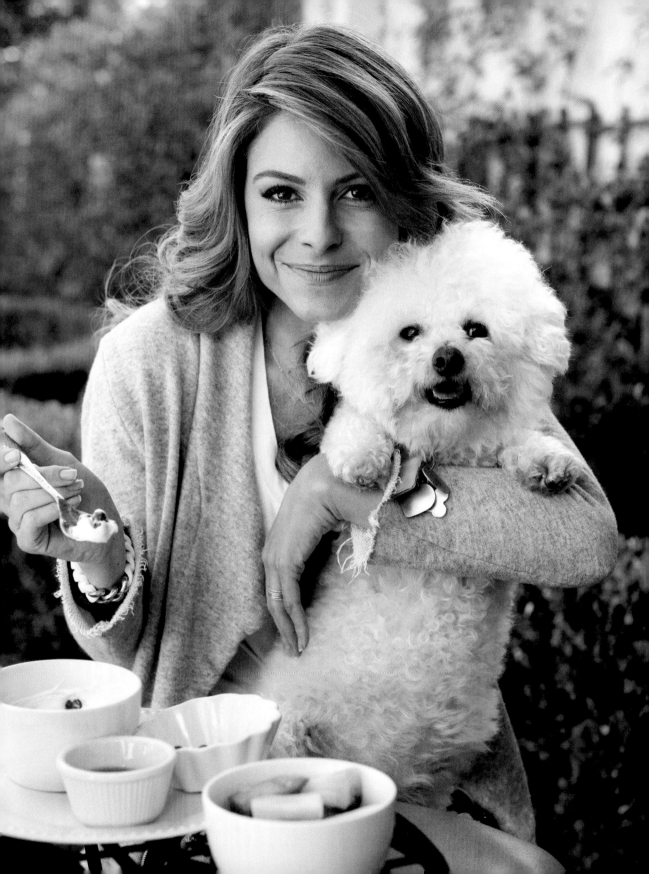

Chapter 6

EveryGirl's Quick Guide to Nutrition and My 75/25 Plan

I don't believe, as I've repeatedly stated, in extreme diet plans—the ones that tell you exactly what to eat and when to eat it, or diets that cut out entire food groups. If I could tell only you two things to help you live a healthier life, they would be that we have been brainwashed to believe we need to eat far more than we legitimately need to. Furthermore, beyond tobacco, alcohol, drugs, and environmental toxins, the type and abundance of food we eat is a key factor in having long-term quality of life.

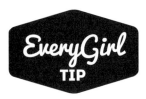

EveryGirl TIP

PROOF ON DIETING
UCLA researchers looked at thirty-one diet studies, and what they found was shocking: Dieting was actually the number one predictor of future weight gain!

Therefore, much of what you read from this point on is the more advanced information I learned in the years following my weight loss. It should all serve you well when engaging in phase 2 of the process.

My 75/25 Plan

One of the ways I maintain my shape and, more important, my health today—and how so many of the friends I turn on to this plan do the same—comes down to one thing: Aim to eat real or whole foods 75 percent of the time. The other 25 percent of the time, you've got room to play.

If all we ate were real or whole foods—fresh fruits, whole grains, chicken, turkey, legumes, nuts, seeds, and vegetables—I doubt any of us would be overweight, and we'd have far fewer health problems, too. People from my dad's village who eat this way often make it to the age of one hundred and beyond. But I personally can't exist *solely* on this, and I bet most of you won't want to either. That's where 75/25 comes in.

Keep in mind the 75/25 plan is a long-term plan for good health, NOT a temporary diet for weight loss. You will lose weight, but, more crucially, you'll be building the foundation for a long and productive life

I'll admit, I sort of backed into this approach. Much of it came from working with Yogi Cameron and from taking the time to understand why my dad has been so successful. So to save you some time and to make losing weight easier, I want to help you create an eating plan that's right for you, using 75/25 as a guide.

Don't Forget Portion Control!

You can eat what you want, but you can't eat as *much* as you want. Whether you're talking about lentils or ice cream, portion control is

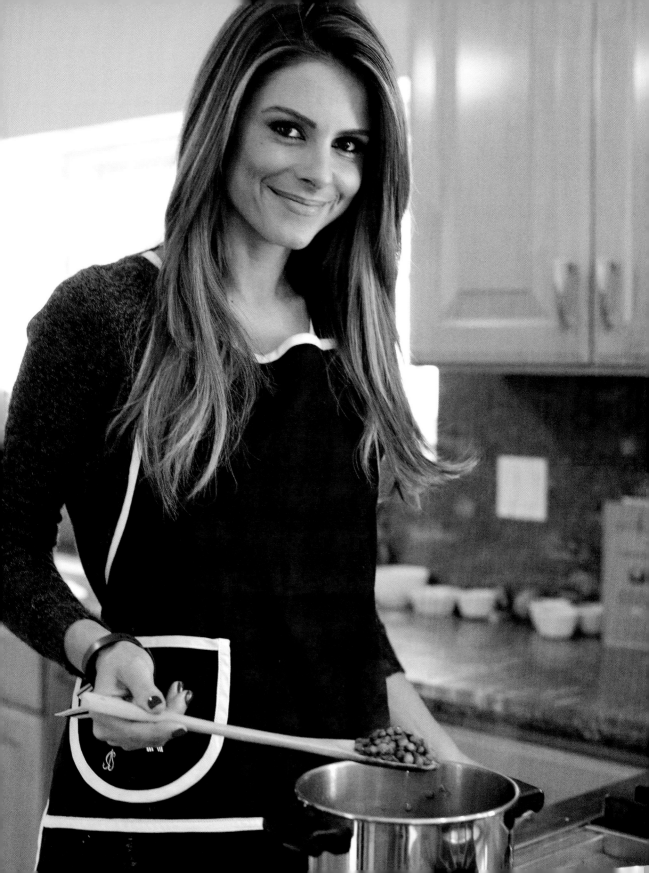

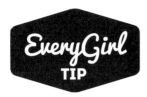

EveryGirl TIP

**PORTION CONTROL...
IS IN THE PALM
OF YOUR HANDS**

Simin Levinson, a lecturer
from the School of Nutrition
and Health Promotion at
Arizona State University,
recommends the best
portion-measuring tool I've
seen: your hands! For protein
like meat, chicken, or fish, she
says the portion should be
able to fit in the palm of your
hand—that is, your palm
minus your fingers and
thumb. For carbs and starch
like potatoes, rice, and pasta,
the portions should be the
size of your fist. Fruit should
fit in one hand, with all five
fingers cupped and rounded.
Vegetables and salads
should fit in two hands,
cupped in the same way.
Cheese should be the size of
your thumb. Oils,
mayonnaise, and other
dressings should match the
tip of your thumb. Make a tall
"C" with your thumb and
forefinger—that's the size of
your glass of fruit juice.
Obviously, this is a rough
guideline, but it's a
convenient and neat way
to assess portions.

important. So when I say eat whatever you want 25 percent of the time, I'm saying eat *sensible portions* of what you want. An ounce or so of chips, not the entire bag. A cup of ice cream, not the entire pint. A slice or two of pizza, not the entire pie. You get the picture. And it's also important not to overdo it on healthy foods. They have calories, too, you know.

What EveryGirl Needs to Know About Nutrition

So which foods should make up the 75 percent of your diet and which ones are 25 percent foods? Knowing a few facts about nutrition will arm you properly in the battle for fitness and health and give you the autonomy to better control your own life and destiny.

Carb Talk

I don't think I'm the only one who's overdone it with carbs. I'd hazard a guess that at least two-thirds of EveryGirl's dietary woes come from over-carbing. But not all carbs are created equal.

All carbs are broken down into glucose (a sugar), which is the fuel your brain and muscles use to keep going. The question is, though, how fast are those carbs digested and converted to glucose? Carbs that are broken down quickly cause all sorts of problems. They give you that quick zap of energy—and then that subsequent crash. They also cause a hormonal imbalance that can cause you to store more of the calories you eat as fat.

One thing that determines how quickly a carb is digested is the amount of fiber in the food. Fiber is the edible part of a plant that does not break down in our stomachs and instead passes through our bodies relatively undigested, absorbing water and easing bowel movements. For practical purposes, that means two things. First, fiber fills you up. Second, it slows the conversion of carbs to glucose. Experts used to talk about the difference between simple carbs (sugar) and complex carbs (starch), but now they're learning that what seems to matter is the amount of *fiber* a carb has. Some simple carbs like fruits and vegetables have fiber and other amazing and essential nutrients, even though the carbs they contain are sugar. Some complex carbs, like white flour, are starches but have very little fiber. They're digested quickly.

Two Types of Fiber

Because fiber is believed to be such a crucial part of health, I'd like to educate you on the two different kinds of fiber:

Insoluble fiber helps to clean out the colon, moving through the digestive system to remove waste and toxins. Since this fiber does not dissolve in water, it passes through your intestines relatively intact, speeding up the passage of food and waste through your gut. Acting like a sponge absorbing

EveryGirl TIP

PORTION CONTOL BAGS
Extra producer, Alina Akram, lost weight by using Ziploc Perfect Portion bags. These single serve bags that prevent freezer burn helped her store her healthy food and manage her portions.

THE HEALTH BENEFITS OF FIBER

→ *Helps control calorie intake. High-fiber foods are often low-calorie foods, and the fiber is also filling.*

→ *Takes a long time to digest. Fibrous foods keep you sated longer.*

→ *Keeps your digestive system healthy and helps to reduce constipation.*

→ *Lowers cholesterol and the risk of heart disease.*

→ *Pulls out excess hormones, fat, and toxins from the body.*

→ *Reduces the risk of certain types of cancer, including colon and breast cancer.*

→ *Reduces high blood pressure.*

water, it also swells inside your stomach and produces a feeling of fullness. Insoluble fibers are mainly found in whole wheat, whole grains, wheat bran, corn bran, seeds, nuts, barley, brown rice, bulgur, zucchini, celery, broccoli, cabbage, onions, tomatoes, carrots, cucumbers, green beans, dark leafy vegetables, raisins, grapes, fruit, and root vegetables.

Soluble fiber attracts water and mixes with digestive enzymes made by the liver; during digestion, it turns to gel. It can bind with harmful substances like excess cholesterol and whisk it out of the body. It's also really filling, so it cuts appetite. Soluble fiber comes from oatmeal, oat cereal, lentils, apples, oranges, grapefruit, pears, oat bran, strawberries, nuts, flaxseeds, beans, barley, dried peas, blueberries, carrots, and psyllium.

When it comes to insoluble and soluble fiber, both are beneficial. How much fiber do you need? Experts say that you should get twenty-five grams of fiber a day, but if you aren't eating much fiber now, you need to increase the amount slowly. If you jump right in, you will likely experience severe gas. Drink plenty of water when you increase your fiber, too.

"Jenny McCarthy shares the same viewpoint as I do when it comes to soup. It works for her, it works for me, and it can work for you. I started eating more soup and pounds melted off me. Soup is filling, low cal, and nutritious."

Tara Kraft, former editor in chief, *Shape* magazine

THE EVERYGIRL'S GUIDE TO DIET AND FITNESS

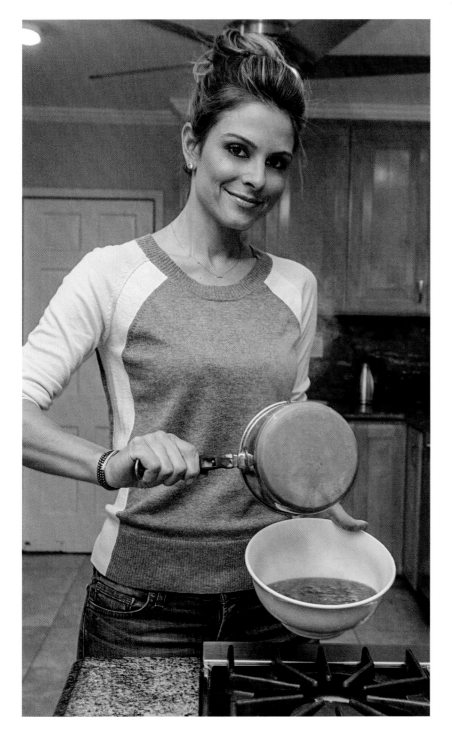

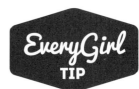

SOUP'S ON!

Another really neat trick for keeping portions in check is to start your meal with a cup of soup. Make it a broth-based one (not cream soups or bisques). They take longer to eat, which is always a good thing, but they are also high in water and low in calories, generally. Studies show that by eating a vegetable-based soup before main meals, you're likely to consume up to 20 percent fewer calories at a meal. Just beware certain canned soups have high sodium levels.

THE GREAT GRAIN DEBATE

Recently, there's been a lot of controversy surrounding grains—are they healthy or harmful? Let's take a look at the arguments on both sides.

The Pro-Grain Argument

Whole grains contain an abundance of nutrients and fiber. They give you a feeling of fullness, motivating you to eat fewer calories and keep a healthy weight. Research shows that people who eat whole-grain diets have healthier weights and gain less over time. Research also shows that diets high in whole grains decrease the risk of diabetes and high blood pressure.

The Anti-Grain Argument

In the first hundred and forty thousand years of human history, grains were not regularly consumed. It's only in the past ten thousand years, when humans went from hunters and gatherers to farmers and harvesters, that we began consuming grains. Some experts assert that humans have not changed much, genetically speaking, in the past ten thousand years and therefore lack the ability to digest and utilize grains, essentially making them a toxin. This opinion is at the center of the Paleolithic or "Paleo" diet that's so popular now. Also known as the caveman or Stone Age diet, it is based only on foods that were available before man turned from hunting and gathering to agriculture. These Paleo diets include fish, grass-fed meats, eggs, vegetables, fruit, fungi, roots, nuts, and healthful oils (olive, walnut, flaxseed, macadamia, avocado, coconut) and exclude grains, legumes, dairy, potatoes, refined salt, refined sugar, and processed oils. Proponents argue that modern human populations who eat this way live longer, healthier lives.

The Gluten Argument

And then there's gluten. I'm sure you've heard of it. It's a protein in wheat and barley that can cause problems for those people with celiac disease or a gluten allergy. And there's the evidence showing that refined grains, in particular, spike insulin levels, which can lead to diabetes and obesity.

I think you should always try to avoid refined grains. As far as whole grains, I think you should eat them. If you have wheat allergies or require a gluten-free diet, you should avoid grains with gluten but eat other whole grains like brown rice, quinoa, and oats.

Good Carbs/Bad Carbs

Here's how to spot the healthy, happiness-giving "good" carbohydrates you should be making a major part of your diet, among the heavy, energy-zapping "bad" ones.

Good Carbs

Legumes. Rich in minerals and low in fat, legumes such as lentils, peas, and beans—such as lima beans, kidney beans, and black beans—are also excellent sources of protein. (Almonds and edamame are legumes as well.)

Whole grains. These contain the germ, endosperm, and bran of the grain, capturing all its nutrients from the ground up. In refined grains the nutrient-rich germ and bran are discarded and only the sugary endosperm is retained. Examples of whole grains include brown rice, quinoa, oats, barley, buckwheat, amaranth, farro, bulgur, einkorn, emmer, and spelt. Eat them in their whole state because when ground into flour, they're digested faster. But pasta, bread, and cereal made from whole grains are okay. Popcorn (skip the butter or the caramel coating) is also a whole grain.

Green vegetables. This includes leafy greens like spinach, lettuce, kale, collards, bok choy, cabbage, and Swiss chard as well as broccoli, Brussels sprouts, green beans, and asparagus.

Other vegetables and fruits like carrots, parsnips, cauliflower, celery, cucumbers, and beets.

Onions, leeks, scallions, and garlic.

Sweet potatoes and winter squash, like butternut or acorn.

Any kind of fruit. However, fruit has more sugar and more calories than vegetables do, so limit yourself to a few pieces a day.

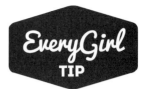

PICK UP GREEN BAGS TO STORE YOUR FRUITS & VEGGIES

Green Bags are food storage bags designed to keep fruits and vegetables crisp and fresh for longer periods of time. There are also reusable plastic green containers for this purpose as well. Check out a brand called Debbie Meyer.

Dried fruit, like raisins, mango, prunes, and apricots. But dried fruit has more calories and sugar per ounce than fresh does, because all the water is gone. So don't go overboard.

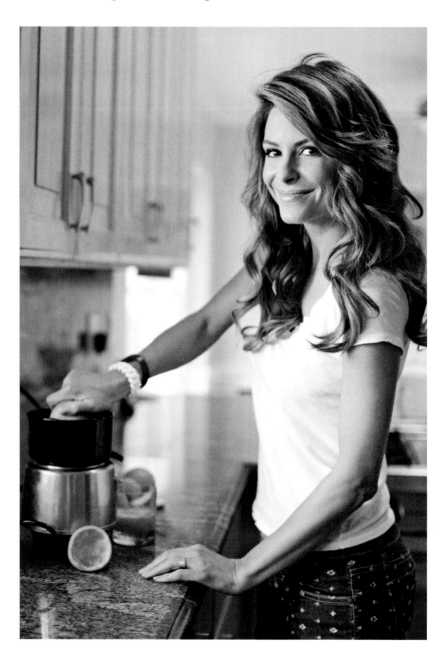

THE EVERYGIRL'S GUIDE TO DIET AND FITNESS

Bad Carbs

Refined grains. These are the ones you want to curb as much as possible, as they turn to sugar quickly after eating. Common refined non-whole grain products include white rice, white flour, white bread, and white pasta.

Sugar. Candy, chocolate, table syrups, anything made with white sugar are all empty calories. Cut back on sugar, and be sure you know all the different names it goes by.

Alcohol.

Fruit juices. Instead of processed fruit juices, eat whole fruit. The nutrients and fiber are great, and whole fruits are slower to digest, leaving you feeling filled up longer. Fresh-squeezed juices like those from Jamba Juice are delicious, and I drink them when I want a special treat. However, important nutrient-rich components such as rinds and pulp are discarded in the squeezing and blending process. Also, since it's a liquid, it's consumed and digested much faster, causing blood sugar levels to spike when consumed on an empty stomach. When you do order fruit juice, be aware that the antioxidants and other phytonutrients in the fruit begin to break down soon after they are exposed to light and air. Therefore, be sure to consume them as soon as they're squeezed. A six to eight-ounce serving is big enough to get your nutrients. Be sure to couple juice with something containing protein to keep blood sugar normal.

Soda. Soda is a big source of sugar in the American diet. Did you know that a twelve-ounce Coke has *nine* teaspoons of sugar in it? Don't get me wrong, I love my occasional Diet Coke, but I normally swap soda for water or skim milk. I know people have a hard time giving up soda. In that case, diet drinks are okay. I'd like to see you limit diet soft drinks. Just remember, juice at least has vitamins and minerals, soda doesn't!

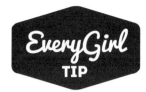

WHAT TO DO ABOUT PASTA

There are conflicting views on pasta. Some say it's not really good for you, that it's high in starch, causes weight gain and quicker energy boosts and dips. Others say it's a decent source of energy, especially when working out. From my research and experience, it's best to opt for whole-wheat pasta when you can. It's rich in fiber and therefore a better, more slowly digested source of energy. However, if that's not available, white pasta is okay—just cut back on the portions, as I did. If one cup of pasta doesn't seem to be filling enough for a meal, extend it by adding some vegetables. If you have a gluten allergy, opt for brown rice pasta or quinoa pasta.

Protein Power

Protein, which is made up of amino acids, builds muscle (with exercise). A pound of muscle burns more calories than a pound of fat does. Protein is also the most satisfying nutrient, which means feeling full on fewer calories. Plus, when you lose weight, unless you take in enough protein, muscle goes first. So you want to get plenty of protein, but just like with carbs, there are good ones and bad ones.

Good Proteins

Lean beef That's beef that has less than ten grams of fat in a $3^1/_2$-ounce serving, such as sirloin, eye of round, top round, and bottom round. Filet mignon is also lean compared to other fancy cuts of beef, but to stay under ten grams of fat, you'd need to eat just three ounces.

Chicken and turkey breast (skinless)

Duck Duck meat is really lean, but remove the fat and skin.

Pork loin and tenderloin

Whitefish, such as haddock, tilapia, grouper, cod, flounder, and sea bass

Salmon

Tuna

Shellfish, such as oysters, clams, shrimp, lobster, mussels, and scallops, as long as they aren't fried

Eggs and egg whites

Nonfat milk

Yogurt, especially Greek yogurt. Plain is best; the flavored ones are often packed with sugar.

Cottage cheese

Low-fat cheeses

Nuts and seeds and nut and seed butter

Tofu and tempeh/soy

Beans and lentils

Bad Proteins

Fatty cuts of beef like prime rib, New York strip, and rib eye

Fried seafood

Full-fat cheese

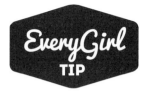

NEVER FATS

Avoid trans fats at all costs. Experts say even a little bit can be damaging to your heart. Look for the words "partially hydrogenated" on ingredients lists of packaged foods. Even if the food label says "No trans fats," if the words "partially hydrogenated" are in the ingredients, then the food contains trans fats. That's because manufacturers can legally say this if the food contains less than half a gram (0.5 grams) of trans fats per serving. But experts say that even just a single gram a day is harmful.

Fabulous Fat

Fat has become a bad word. We don't like to eat fat because we don't want to be fat. But fat doesn't make you fat. Too many junk calories, no matter where they come from, are what make people fat. And the fact is that we need fat—healthy fat. It's not only good for such things as brain development, but it also keeps us satiated. So don't shy away, make sure to include some throughout the day—whether it's an avocado or extra-virgin olive oil (make your own salad dressing with it and vinegar), for example. I also love a little coconut milk. Just make sure to make best efforts to avoid the "bad" fats that exist.

Good Fats

Avocado

Nuts and seeds, and nut and seed butters

Oils like olive, walnut, hazelnut, canola

Coconut oil

Olives

Bad Fats

Butter

Whole milk

Cream

Full-fat cheeses like Cheddar

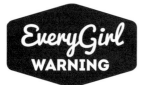

EveryGirl WARNING

FANCY NAMES FOR SUGAR

As consumers grow wise to the detriments of sugar, manufacturers are stepping up their game to combat it by using other names for it. Here is a list for you to be aware of:

Agave nectar

Brown sugar

Cane crystals

Cane sugar

Corn sweetener

Corn syrup

Crystalline fructose

Dextrose

Evaporated cane juice

Organic evaporated cane juice

Fructose

Fruit juice concentrates

Glucose

High-fructose corn syrup

Honey

Invert sugar

Lactose

Maltose

Malt syrup

Molasses

Raw sugar

Sucrose

Syrup

RESIST SUGAR

America consumes nearly twenty times the amount of sugar it did two hundred years ago, just as we are hearing more and more that sugar could possibly be the worst and most destructive ingredient for your health. It has virtually no nutrients, and worse, it's in practically everything most of us eat.

Some people, such as those with high metabolisms, quickly burn sugar off as energy. However, more often, people end up storing sugar as fat and thus gaining weight. Excess sugar leads to obesity, diabetes, cardiovascular disease, dementia, macular degeneration, renal failure, chronic kidney disease, high blood pressure, and maybe cancer.

If that doesn't impress you, then let me appeal to your vanity. Sugar will age you more rapidly and show on your face as well as your waistline and body. It taxes your body harshly and also leads to mood swings. I love my candy, especially sour candy, as well as my ice cream and dessert. I don't think I'd be able to cut it out. However, preparing this book has inspired me to cut back all over again. I hope you can do the same.

Beware of High-Fructose Corn Syrup

High-fructose corn syrup is extracted from corn, and it's sweeter than regular sugar. It is cheaper to make than regular sugar, so food manufacturers use it in a lot. It's in soda, cereal, yogurt, candy, ketchup, spaghetti sauce—so many things! There's a lot of controversy surrounding this sweetener. Some say it's the same as sugar, but more and more evidence shows that it's different. High-fructose corn syrup and sugar both contain fructose. The only organ that can metabolize fructose is the liver; as you may know, the liver is an organ you do not want to mess with. There's also some evidence that high-fructose corn syrup makes you fatter than regular sugar. In a controlled experiment with two groups of rats, the rats that were fed high-fructose corn syrup gained significantly more weight than those that were fed table sugar.

128

Get Started

So there you have it—easy to follow nutrition guidelines that you can use throughout your (long, healthy) life, not just while losing weight. You can now start playing around with the 75/25 approach and begin putting together meals that appeal to you. In the next chapter, I share additional tips for losing weight and keeping it off. But I want to end this chapter by reminding you that you don't have to be rigid with the 75/25 plan. You can also decide that you want to do an 80/20 plan or a 90/10 plan, or maybe even a 60/40 or 50/50 plan. These are simply guidelines to help you create the plan that will work for you.

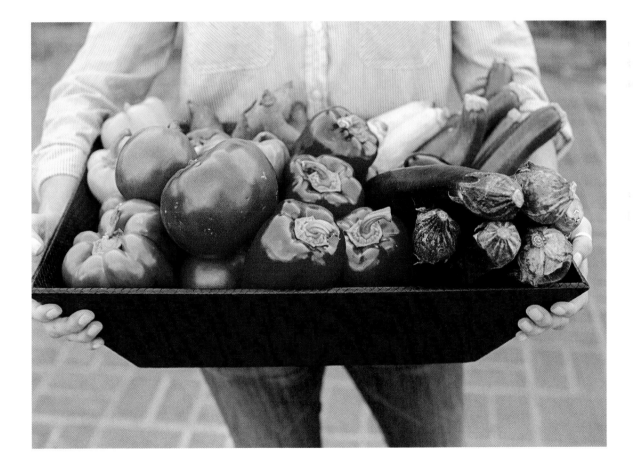

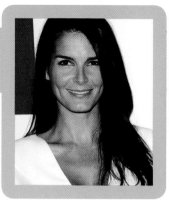

What is your philosophy on weight loss?

We get only one body. If we're blessed and healthy, it's our job to keep it that way. Life is a beautiful thing, and I want to be here for a long time. It's crucial to take care of yourself: to eat the right foods, to workout, to take care of your skin and hair, to sleep well, to take care of your mind.

What are your favorite pre- and post-workout foods?

You need carbs for your brain to function. Before a workout I'll have a snack like yogurt with cereal. It's easy on my digestive system and gives me energy for a great workout, without a ton of calories. Afterwards, I'll have a protein bar. But those can get tricky, and you have to look at the label. If the carbs are greater than the protein, it's a glorified candy bar.

What's one food people should remove from their diets?

Sodium. I love it. I love a good Bloody Mary. I love a huge plate of nachos. I love that stuff, but when I wake up the next morning my face is so puffy. I look like I'm having an allergic reaction, and it's not just my face. As soon as I dial down my sodium intake, my jeans are more comfortable and I just feel better.

What does your workout routine consist of?

I like to workout in the morning so I'm on a high for the rest of the day. My personal program is high cardio, but I also incorporate Pilates to shape my legs and rear end.

What body-image issues do you share with the EveryGirl?

I think we're all trying to keep up with life and stay ahead of the game; and we all have our imperfections. We all have something that we're continuously working on.

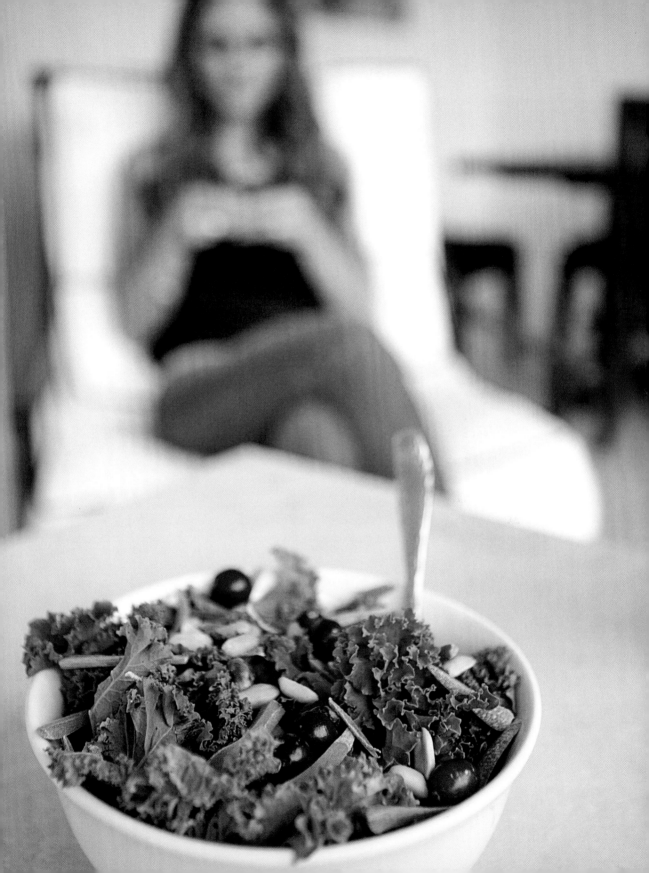

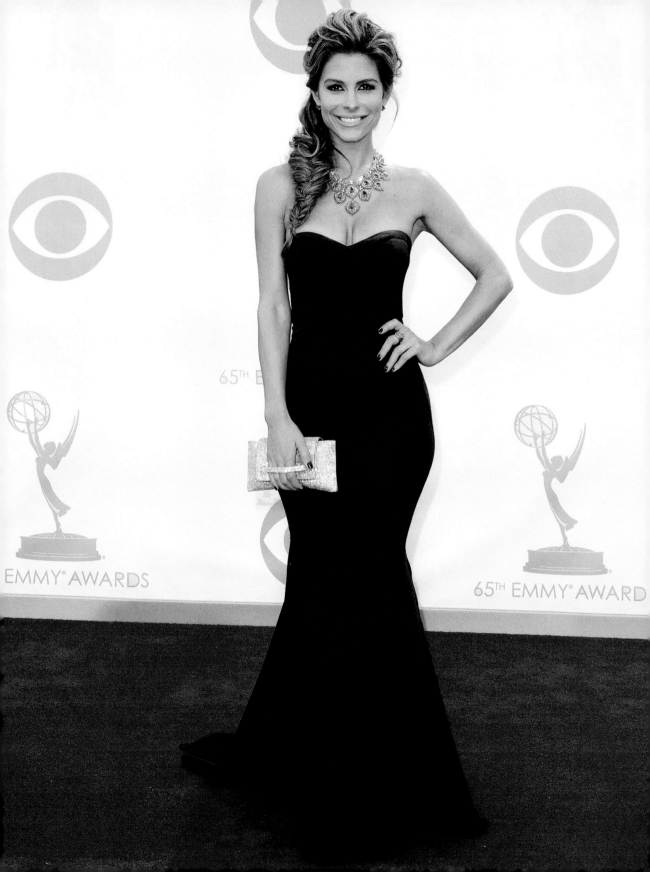

Chapter 7

EveryGirl's Tips and Tricks to Keeping It Off

By now you've gone through the 13 steps to weight loss, and following the 75/25 plan has become second nature. But that doesn't mean you'll stay at exactly the same weight for the rest of your life. Even though I've successfully kept the bulk of the weight off for more than twelve years, my weight does fluctuate from time to time. I've also had some health ups and downs that have, in one way or another, affected my diet. But when my weight goes up, I return to the strategies in the previous two chapters, and I also double up on the following strategies.

The "Best" Way to Eat

There's a lot of disagreement about the healthiest way to eat. Some people tell you to have small meals throughout the day and others

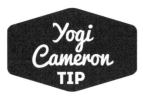

YOGI CAMERON TIP

YOU DON'T NEED 3–4 SET MEALS A DAY

Yogi Cameron doesn't believe it's necessary to have a number of established meals per day. He references yogis in India who eat only enough to sustain themselves, and yet are active and working at the age of 100.

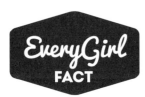

EVERYGIRL FACT

LONG LIVE UNPROCESSED EATS

Cultures that boast the most centarians (those who live to be 100 years old, or older!) have one thing in common: Their diets consist mainly of unprocessed foods. Stick with foods that come from the ground and you could live past 100, too!

→ These were my daily reminders on my kitchen corkboards during the stress rash days.

say three square meals. You have to be a vegetarian–no, you have to have meat in your diet. Breakfast is the most important meal of the day–no, it's okay to skip it. The bottom line is that you simply have to do what's right for your body and your lifestyle. Yogi Cameron has three basic principles that I swear by and believe will be helpful to you:

EAT MOSTLY FOODS THAT COME FROM THE GROUND.
EAT ONLY WHEN YOU ARE HUNGRY.
EAT ONLY AS MUCH AS YOU NEED IN THE MOMENT.

Let's look at these points one by one:

Eat mostly foods that come from the ground. I mentioned this in my EveryGirl Rules to Live By, but want to expand on it now. When I was suffering with my rash, Yogi Cameron told me to eat fresh fruits, vegetables, legumes, nuts, seeds, and whole grains–anything that came from a plant. This was simple, clean food that was easy for my body to absorb nutrients from. Making this simple dietary change prevented the rash from spreading and allowed my body's defenses to better combat it. If I had the willpower, I would exclusively eat food from the ground. The prob-

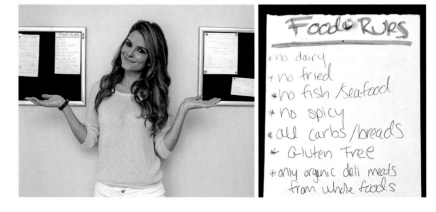

THE EVERYGIRL'S GUIDE TO DIET AND FITNESS

lem is that I love eating and love some processed foods. That said, I just do my best and often rotate my diet plan depending on my life and health status at any given time, and I use this notion as my healthy barometer. The time I get really serious about it is when I think I'm getting sick or even just when I'm feeling polluted from a long spell of bad eating. You know, those times when you just eat and drink horribly for a while, like during the holidays or a vacation. There are Mondays after certain weekends I feel this way, too. By eating foods from the ground and drinking lots of water, my body feels cleansed and refreshed.

Eat only when hungry. I wrote this quote of Cameron's down and hung it on my corkboard as a daily reminder. As I've said, we don't need nearly as much food as we think we do. "More is more" has become a cultural staple, and our restaurant portions are proof. You'll be amazed at how little you really need every day when you consciously attempt eating less.

Try eating based on the signals you're getting from your body. It may take a little time to get in tune with them. But once you do, you'll discover that some days, you may not be hungry in the morning, and other days, you may feel famished as soon as you wake up. Let your body guide you.

One day, as an experiment, I decided to listen to my body's natural hunger cues, and I found that I wasn't hungry until 1:30 p.m. At that point, I had a handful of blueberries and realized, hmmm, my stomach seems satisfied, let me find out what it tells me next. I remember sometime around five o'clock, I got hungry again. I then ate some grilled chicken and a sweet potato. That was it for the day.

I don't eat that way every day, of course. Most of the time, I eat three meals a day and occasionally have a snack. That just seems to fit in with my family, work, and schedule, but I try my best to eat only what I need within those meals.

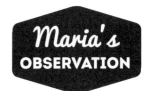

Maria's OBSERVATION

I used to say to myself, "I'm going to load up on a big meal now because I may not have the time to eat later." I did believe that, but it was really my excuse to overeat. The reality is you'll always find the time and means to get the food you need. Just eat what your body requires, and eat when you're hungry.

Eat only as much as you need. You can also check in with your body mid-meal to see how full you are so that you can stop eating before you stuff yourself. When you feel full, listen to what your body is telling you and then put down your fork, no matter how good the food tastes.

As I advised earlier, take eating breaks during meals. Halfway through, stop eating for a few minutes to get up and walk to the bathroom, for example. The break gives your brain a chance to register that your stomach is getting full and let you know that it's close to quitting time.

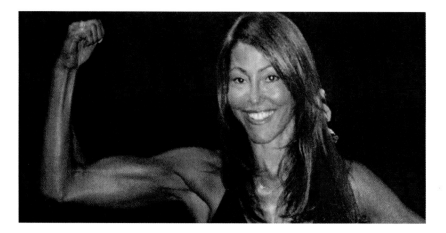

→ Though she's RIPPED in this photo, she also looks very feminine when not flexing!!!

The Tale of Deb Silverstein

One of my friends, Deb Silverstein, has a rock-solid body and beautiful skin. She looks like she's in her thirties, but she is really in her fifties. I know that only because her husband and my old boss at *Access Hollywood,* Rob Silverstein, told me. And the only reason he did is because he is that proud of her. Deb hasn't had any cosmetic surgery or other similar enhancements. She merely eats right and exercises. One time, Kev and I were hiking with Deb and Rob and the subject of weight loss, workouts, and diets came up. Rob, Kev, and

I all weighed in on the subject. When it was Deb's turn, she shrugged and said, "When it comes to keeping weight off or weight loss, it really just comes down to eating less."

There are exceptions, of course—people with genetic disorders, for instance—but generally, it's true. Just as eating things grown from the ground will help you live a healthy life, the simple act of eating less is the best and surest way to lose weight or prevent weight gain.

Eating clean, like Deb does, not only keeps her in great shape, but keeps her looking young by preventing wrinkles. Her food choices keep her organs healthy, and skin is the body's largest organ. Deb Silverstein, like my dad, is on the fifty-year plan to diet and fitness. The results speak for themselves. Personally, I don't have Deb's discipline, or her body, but she gives us all something to aspire to.

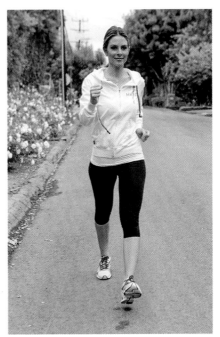

Use Smaller Plates

If you use large plates, you're more likely to want to fill that plate—and thus eat more. Many experts recommend that you downsize your dishes to help trick yourself into thinking (and thus feeling) as if you've eaten more than you have. While it may not be the only answer, it can give you a mental boost, which is especially helpful when you're starting to cut portion sizes. It totally works for me.

Make Dinner the Smallest Meal of the Day

This is tough, because traditionally this is the biggest meal of the day. But the fact that you'll be in bed in a few hours and have less time to burn those calories off is a good reason to keep dinner smaller. And while you're at it:

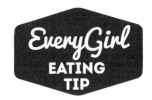

Take smaller bites and chew food thoroughly. This will help you to eat more slowly, giving you more time to fill up. It also allows you to absorb more nutrients and energy from your food. In addition, chewing longer makes food easier to digest.

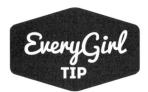

WATER FILTERS

I had my dad install inexpensive water filters on my kitchen and bathroom sinks. My water is pure and clean tasting, and having it so easily accessible makes me more likely to drink it. Built-in filters also eliminate the bulk, expense, and inconvenience of buying bottled water.

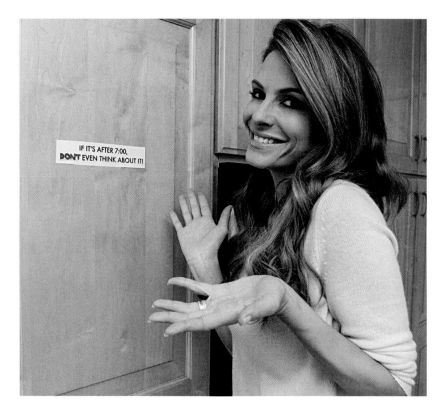

CHIP SWAP

Try baby carrots sprinkled with sea salt when you're craving something crunchy. Carrots also take longer to chew than chips do, and have more fiber (to fill you up!), so they're a healthy way to curb your hunger.

Try Not to Eat After 7 p.m.

For years I was a restless sleeper, and my body would get really hot at night and I'd sweat like crazy. Cameron taught me that eating late in the evening, especially spicy foods (which I love), was causing this. The heat came from the spicy foods but also because my body was still digesting my meal while I was sleeping.

Nowadays, I have dinner before 7:30 p.m. If, by chance, I get home later and am hungry, I will eat something small and clean, like Greek yogurt with blueberries. That's also what I go for if I'm up late and I get hungry. It usually takes the edge off and feels like a dessert at the same time. Other times, if I'm hungry late at night, Kev will tell me to just "sleep it off." When I do, I wake up feeling fine, and I'm no more hungry than I am on any other morning.

Think of Food As Fuel

Start seeing food as something that will energize your body, not satisfy your taste buds. When you think about food this way, rather than a source of pleasure, it's much easier to choose the salad with grilled chicken instead of the burger melt. And remember, for better results over the long term, you want your body to run on high-quality fuel, so give it as much unprocessed fare as you can.

BEST WAYS TO FILL UP AND FEEL FULL

Load up on veggies and salad. They have a lot of water and fiber, which fill you up for very few calories. For the calories in just one little cheese cube, you could have four entire cups of cherry tomatoes.

Eat protein at every meal because it keeps you full for hours.

Don't have carb-only meals, because your blood sugar will spike and then drop, increasing your cravings for more carbs. You'll be hungry all the time!

Keep a small bag of almonds in your bag or in your desk. They'll take the edge off when you're starving, and they'll keep you away from "bad" snacks or fast food.

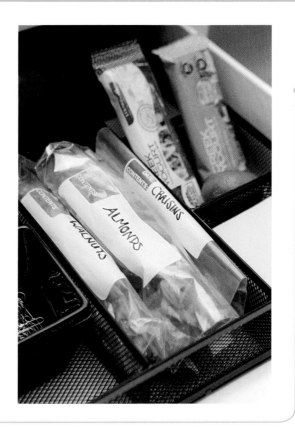

Drink Lots of Water—Room Temperature and Hot

I'm repeating myself because drinking water, particularly hot water, has been such a game-changer for me. I start my day with hot water, and I have electric kettles from Target in my kitchen and my office so that I can drink it throughout the day as well. Sometimes I like my water room temperature or cold, so I can have that instead of a drink with tons of calories.

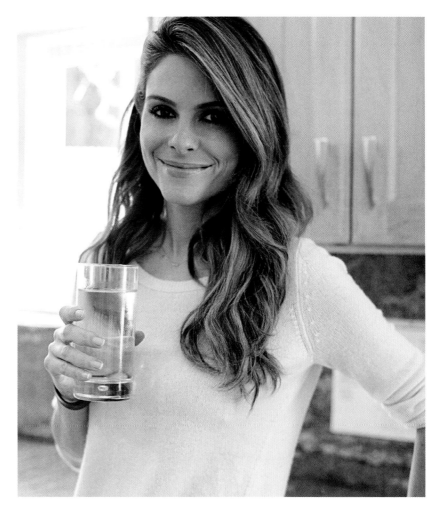

Once you get in the habit of drinking water throughout the day, you'll be amazed at the increase in energy levels and the decrease in hunger levels you'll experience. And some studies even show that people who drink two glasses of water before meals lose more weight and kept it off compared to those who don't.

Poor Health: Emotions Initiate It, Food Exacerbates It

I'm convinced that my rash was caused by stress and that many ailments are due to emotions. And the food choices you make can either help cure illness, or they can exacerbate it. In the future when you're sick, take the time to consider how your dietary choices may be affecting your overall health.

Cope with Cravings

When a craving hits, it's helpful to be able to tell the difference between actually being hungry and boredom, or some other emotion. If your craving is due to hunger, give in with something healthy. Looking at your food journal should make you aware of the times you tend to reach for candy or a snack during your day. Once you notice a pattern, you can make sure that you do something else during that time. Try going for a quick stroll outside or even through your office. And grab a hot water while you're at it.

It's smart to choose a healthy emergency food that you like—one that's low-cal, that can satisfy cravings—and to always have it on hand. I suggest that you choose something crunchy, like raw veggies, because they can give you the feeling of a chip fix without the chips.

Having a small bag of almonds on hand is amazing, too. Almonds are high in fiber and protein and will fill you up. You might hear people tell you that they're fattening, but I assure you that in

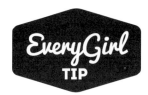

HOLIDAY EATING

There is no way I'm ever going to advise you to cut back on holiday eating, because it's literally my favorite time of year to cook and to eat! However, I've heard of families who work out the morning of holidays and other people who play sports like tag football. Last year I engaged in a "Dance War" with my holiday guests. When Derek and Julianne Hough caught wind, they did the same, and soon we had an Instagram video battle. My guests and I danced so much that I was sore the next day. It was a fun way to burn off some holiday treats.

Another trick I use around holiday time is to cut back a bit the week before and the week after. Small cutbacks help you enjoy the holidays guilt-free.

moderation they are not. Scientists in Australia had a group of people add about one and a half ounces of almonds to their diets every day and had others eat the way they normally would for a month. You'd think that the people eating nuts would get heavier, right? But that's not what happened. They didn't gain any weight, probably because the almonds were so satisfying that they unconsciously ate less of other foods.

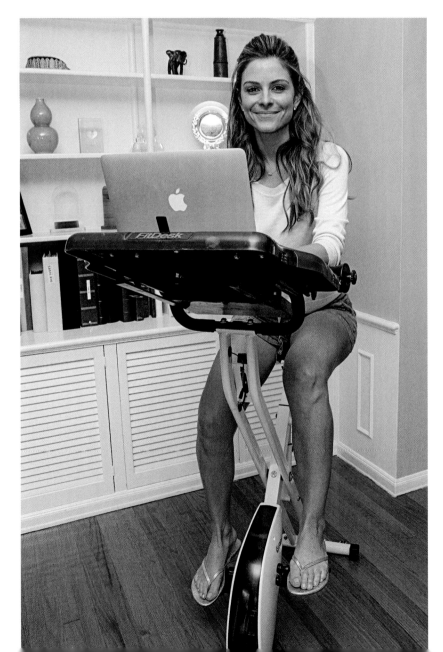

↗ I really love this FitDesk P.S. No one is paying me to say this (or anything else in this book, by the way). It will run you about $299, and if you have a home office it's a great way to do two things at once. And it's actually comfortable. I do it, then shower with baby wipes!! Make it work!

Earn Your Food

When I know I'm going to eat poorly later in the day, say hitting one of my favorite Italian restaurants where I plan to heavily indulge, I tell myself I have to "earn" those foods. On those days I'm more physically active, moving with an even higher energy level than I normally do. I engage in as much activity as possible, and consciously try to earn the right to eat those less-than-healthy foods later in the day. Another way I earn my indulgences is by using a FitDesk, a stationary bike with a built-in desk that I can put my laptop on. I work while pedaling and burning extra calories. I do it for a few minutes here and there while returning e-mails. I have friends who have desk attachments on their treadmills, too.

Take Ultimate Control— and Learn to Cook

I loved cooking for my family when my parents had to work late, and I still enjoy cooking today. (In chapter 8, I supply you with twenty-two easy and delicious recipes that my family and I eat all the time.) When you know your way around the kitchen, *you* get to decide what goes into your food, and that means you can keep calories down and healthy nutrients up. Fortunately, you don't have to go to culinary school in order to cook healthy meals. With all the cookbooks and YouTube videos out there, there are plenty of ways to learn how to cook quick, healthy meals. Maybe there's someone in your family who likes to cook and can teach you, or maybe you have a friend who is also interested in learning how to cook. Classes are more fun with friends. If you're really savvy, you can get a few friends to pitch in and hire a chef for a group lesson. It's a fun night out and a healthy use of your time.

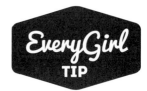

TRY NOT TO EAT IN FRONT OF THE TV

Some studies indicate that you consume more salt or sugar when you eat in front of the TV because your mind is so focused on watching that it needs stronger flavors to register with your brain. That's not good for maintaining weight loss! The same can be said for eating while surfing the Web or while driving.

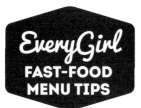

EveryGirl FAST-FOOD MENU TIPS

Salad, veggie burger, or grilled chicken sandwich at Burger King

———

Salad, grilled chicken sandwich, or grilled chicken wrap at McDonald's

———

Fresco-style items at Taco Bell

———

Grilled chicken sandwich and baked potato at Wendy's

———

A sandwich made with lean meat, like turkey or ham, and a lot of veggies at Subway. You can ask them to scoop out the inside of the bread, or you can even have them toss everything into a salad instead of having a sandwich. I grab a quick bite at Subway all the time.

Stock Your Kitchen Right

Fact: You're only as good an eater as your environment allows. What does that mean? If you have a pantry full of chips, you're going to eat those chips. If they're not there, you won't eat them. It sounds simple, but every time there was junk food in my cabinets, chances are I ended up eating it. Everything in your fridge, cabinets, and desk drawers should be healthy and nutritious.

What's in my fridge?

- Greek yogurt
- Fuji apples
- Blueberries
- Skim milk
- Salad mix
- Broccoli
- Carrots
- Hummus
- Vanilla ice cream
- Any healthy meals I've cooked up for the week

Be Smart When Eating Out

Frequently dining at restaurants makes it hard to keep the weight off. The portions are huge; there are all those extras, like the bread basket; and chefs tend to use a lot of butter and oil in their cooking (and salt, too). That said, there are many things you can do to make sure that restaurant meals don't pack on the pounds. One of the best strategies is to ask for steamed vegetables as a side dish instead of carb-heavy ones. Always ask for no butter because restaurants often use butter to make vegetables taste richer and look shiny and appetizing. No matter how much you want to say yes to the fries or mashed potatoes, just ask for vegetables or a salad with oil and vinegar (on the side, always). Eventually this will become second nature. If you're thinking there is no way you can do this, then you're exactly like I was when I started. Once you get through Phase One and start seeing those positive results, it will get easier. Trust me!

You can even eat healthily at fast-food places. I'd love for all of us to eat nothing but fruits, vegetables, legumes, and grains plucked from our own backyards, but that's not realistic. Sometimes fast food is the only option because it is inexpensive or because you need something, well, fast. Sometimes, such as when you're in an airport, fast food is the only option available. Fortunately, you don't have to resort to a burger and fries. More and more fast-food restaurants are offering healthy menu options to help you get by.

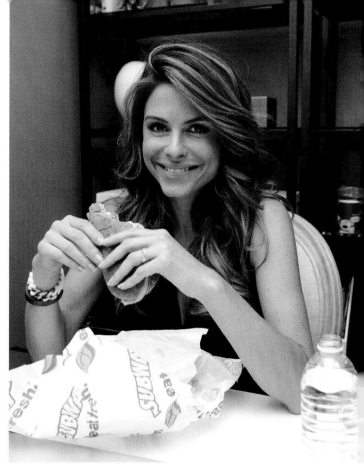

"If it's not rude, I try to order first because the first order influences the rest of the table. If someone orders something decadent, it lets you off the hook and you think, 'What the hell!'"

Michele Promaulayko, editor in chief, *Women's Health* magazine

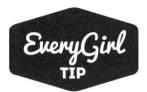

EveryGirl TIP

If you're going out with friends and know everyone will be pigging out at dinner, and you won't be able to resist, plan to meet them for after-dinner drinks or coffee instead of the entire meal.

Schedule Something Else for Your Lunch Hour

If your coworkers like going to unhealthy places for lunch, it may be best to bow out, even if it seems antisocial. Instead, eat something light at your desk before taking a walk or getting in a quick workout. I use this tactic because my colleagues are often eating hot dogs, fries, and other foods that aren't ideal. If I'm with them, I'm much more liable to say, "Screw it" and join them. If I stay at my desk, never smell the food, and stay focused, I'm not tempted and I don't know what I've missed! One step closer to my goal.

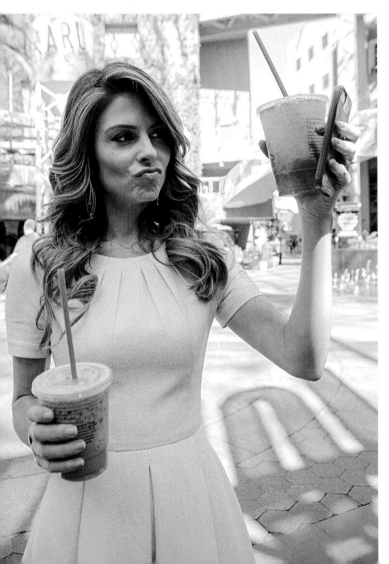

Swap Out Your Vices

So many people fall into the trap of having a certain unhealthy food or drink every day. They do it out of habit, without even thinking. But maybe if they stopped to think about it, they'd realize there's a healthier option that they'd enjoy just as much. Drinking soda or diet soda is one example. Consider replacing soda with green tea. It may not be easy at first, but it won't take too long for you to adjust.

Hang Out with Healthy Eaters

I mentioned this when I talked about building a healthy foundation. Here's how it worked out for me. On a recent trip to Greece with our friends Marietta and Leon, we ate healthily because Marietta is all about fresh food and because the portions are smaller there. If Kev and I hadn't been with them the whole trip, I definitely would have splurged and come back home heavier and more exhausted. I have so many great friends who eat poorly, and I'm not about to dump them for it. However, if you are trying to get in shape, just be aware that their company may not be the best thing in certain situations.

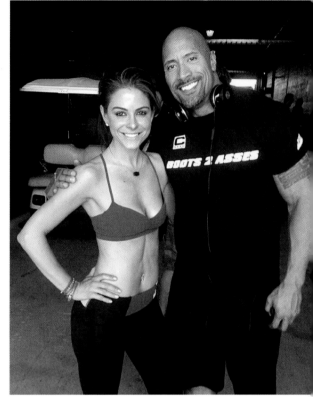

↑ Here I am at WrestleMania with my friend Dwayne Johnson, aka the Rock. I love reading his tweets because they inspire me to work out, although I don't know if I'll ever be able to do the 4 a.m. workout like him. But he did inspire me to do the 6:30 a.m. workout once in a while.

Curbing the EveryGirl Sweet Tooth

If refined sugars are your weak spot, as carbs were mine, try these tips.

➜ Look at your journal and determine when you are most likely to reach for sugar. Also consider how you were feeling when you got a sugar craving. Were you stressed, happy, tired, bored?

➜ Once you figure out when and why you are consuming sugar, then find another activity to do the next time you get a craving: Exercise, reach out to a friend, walk, drink hot water, or have raw veggies and protein to make you feel full.

➜ Swap high-sugar foods for low-sugar foods. Instead of having soda after work, maybe have green tea. If you really want something sweet, try fruit or, interestingly enough, dark chocolate. Neither one will spike your blood sugar levels, so they won't make you crash after you eat them. Look for dark chocolate—it should have a cocoa

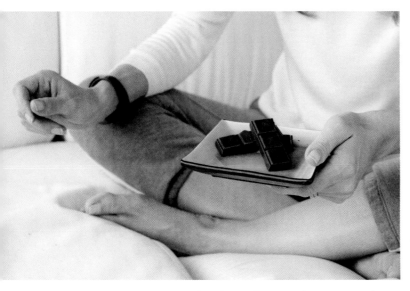

content of 70 percent or more. And FYI, dark chocolate has much less sugar than milk chocolate.

➔ Don't keep sugary items at home, in your bag, in your car, or in your desk. No need to tempt yourself unnecessarily.

➔ Scale back sugars *slowly*, just as we did with other foods. If you drink six sodas every day, have five tomorrow. The next day, have four, and so on until you are having only one—or none.

➔ If you are going to eat sugar, have it before your workout. That gives you a greater chance of burning the sugar and carbs as energy instead of storing them as fat.

One thing that helps me to avoid sugar is thinking about the inevitable crash from it later. I splurge on sugar at times, but knowing how a sugar crash will disrupt my day is a great means to dissuade me.

Grow Your Own Food

Having a garden of your own is fun, rewarding, cost efficient, convenient, and healthy. You don't need a lot of money to plant a garden. My mom and dad did it when they were poor. I once did a TV segment with a great company called Gro-O, which specializes in teaching people how to start an organic garden at home. Their representatives came to my house and taught me how to plant a garden of my own. We installed two four-foot by eight-foot planters in my backyard, filled them with soil, and planted tomatoes, cucumbers,

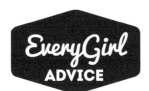

EveryGirl ADVICE

TEACH YOUR KIDS HEALTHY HABITS

Get children on the right track—eating foods from the ground and avoiding sugar and refined carbs—from an early age. Sugar addiction is built up over time, so this is crucial. My parents had me eating food grown from the ground ever since I was born. It's how I was raised, and, even though I strayed in college, the diet I was reared on was permanently ingrained in my taste buds. That's what made it so easy and natural for me to resume it.

zucchini, eggplants, basil, garlic, carrots, cantaloupe, and more. In a few months, I had all this healthy food right outside my door. I was so inspired that I started cooking more.

Before I had the garden, I'd work until I was starving, then be forced to go out to eat. Now I can whip up a variety of delicious, healthy meals very easily. You can't get higher-octane fuel for your body than fresh, pesticide-free produce. The garden's great for my wallet, too, as I eat out less and make fewer trips to the supermarket.

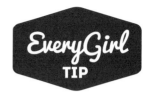

HATCH YOUR OWN EGGS
Do you have room to raise chickens? If so, consider raising some to yield farm-fresh eggs. My parents' neighbors in Connecticut do.

EVERYGIRL CAN HAVE A GARDEN

If you live in an apartment, plant your favorite veggies in pots and keep them on the balcony.

No balcony, or you live in a cold climate? Try planting at least a few fresh herbs in a window box and put it on a sunny windowsill.

Some cities have community gardens where you can get a plot to plant and harvest your own crops. Look into one near you.

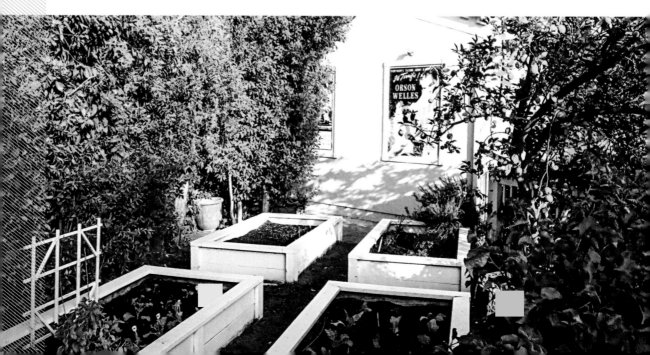

Let's be honest: We all want to live long lives and have a good quality of life at the same time, but we also want to look great, too. Our facial skin is so incredibly delicate compared to the skin on other areas of our bodies. Poor diet, especially too much sugar, affects it, but so do many other factors.

Cigarette Smoking

I'm surprised that for all the money anti-smoking campaigns shell out, they've never hit on the one essential thing I think would motivate people, especially women, to quit smoking—or never even start: Cigarettes severely age and ravage your face!

I'm a huge movie buff, and I particularly love watching the old movies shown on Turner Classic Movies. I've seen many of my favorite old movie stars—who worked in an era when smoking was not only popular, but encouraged—age drastically over the course of their careers. Here's a peek at what's in store for you if you smoke.

PALE, WORN-OUT SKIN: Smoking deprives skin of oxygen and other nutrients, leaving smokers' faces pale and drawn out.

SUN SPOTS: Smokers are far more susceptible to them.

SAGGING SKIN: According to the American Lung Association there are approximately 600 ingredients in cigarettes that, when burned, create more than 4,000 chemicals. Chemicals that trigger the destruction of collagen and elastin—the proteins that give your skin strength and elasticity. This causes sagging in your face and other areas of your body, like your arms and breasts.

WRINKLES: Pursing your lips to draw on the cigarette over and over again, combined with the loss of skin elasticity, will create deep lines around your mouth. Smokers are also more likely to have very noticeable crow's feet around their eyes.

YELLOW TEETH: Maybe you think you can whiten them, but smokers are twice as likely to lose teeth and to have persistent gum and breath problems.

WEAK BONES: What does this have to do with your looks? If osteoporosis sets in, you could develop an arched back.

OTHER ISSUES: Besides cancer and heart and lung issues, smoking also contributes to psoriasis, infertility, cataracts, and early menopause.

Alcohol

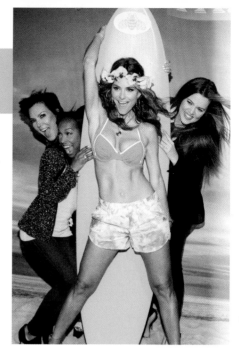

I enjoy drinking occasionally, but the truth is, I rarely do. Moderate drinking can be good for you. It helps lower cholesterol and reduces the risk of heart attack, dementia, and even diabetes, because it improves the body's sensitivity to insulin. That said, when done to excess, there are destructive effects. It raises the risk of liver damage, breast cancer, depression, and more. And it has a negative impact on your looks.

WRINKLES: Like smoking, too much alcohol causes premature wrinkles due to a loss of collagen and elasticity.

RUDDY COMPLEXION: Alcohol is a vasodilator, meaning that it widens the blood vessels that bring blood to the face, causing puffiness or swelling. This may lead to permanent redness and blotchy skin as well as broken capillaries.

DEHYDRATION: Alcohol is a diuretic. The more you drink, the more dehydrated you get. Dehydrating your body and especially your skin is incredibly damaging. Follow each drink with a glass of water. It helps avoid hangovers, drinking water in between drinks keeps you (and your skin) hydrated.

Recreational Drugs

Drugs will ravage your face as much as alcohol and smoking, but that's the least of it. I see so many people on pills (prescription or otherwise) who are short-tempered, off-kilter, extremely emotional, negative, depressed, lazy or overcome by dark emotions. Most don't even realize it. Like so many people in our country, they're stressed or in pain and choose to ease it with pills, treating the symptom and not the problem.

Drugs will age you and also destroy you. Take all possible steps to avoid them, and if you are using them, please get help. There are professionals you can reach out to.

Maria's Seven-Day Food Journal

Here's what a recent seven-day stretch looked like for me. I'm not perfect, as you can see, but I aim for a 75-25.

	BREAKFAST	LUNCH	DINNER	SNACKS & SIPS
SUN	Greek yogurt with blueberries; hot water with lemon	Turkey wrap with provolone cheese, lettuce, onion, and mustard	2 small slices cheese pizza and a small order of cheese ravioli in Alfredo sauce	Hot water
MON	Harley Pasternak's White Breakfast Smoothie (apple, banana, Greek yogurt, almonds, and milk); hot water with lemon	Salad made with chicken, tomato, onion, Feta, and a vinaigrette dressing	Chili's nachos, loaded potato skins, and a small garden salad (no cheese)	Hot water with lemon
TUES	2 scrambled egg whites with spinach and a side of mixed fruit; hot water with lemon	Harley Pasternak's Red Smoothie (orange juice, raspberries, blueberries, milk, flaxseed, and protein powder)	Greek salad with chicken	Twizzlers, Diet Coke, and hot water with lemon
WED	Harley Pasternak's White Breakfast Smoothie; hot water with lemon	Turkey sandwich with avocado and cheese; side salad	Skirt steak panini with side salad	Nonfat iced hazelnut latte; hot water with lemon
THURS	Harley Pasternak's White Breakfast Smoothie; hot water with lemon	2 slices of white pesto pizza and a side salad	Mom's mixed vegetables (recipe on page 158) with chicken	Hot water with lemon
FRI	2 scrambled egg whites with spinach; hot water with lemon	Greek salad with chicken	Gyro with tzatziki sauce; 2 of Mom's Baked Breaded Zucchini patties (recipe on page 162)	Hot water with lemon
SAT	French toast; hot water with lemon	Salad (with vegetables from my garden) with avocado, corn, chicken, carrots	Sushi: 3 baked crab hand rolls and a spicy tuna roll; edamame; 2 green tea mochi ice cream treats	Iced coffee with skim milk and sugar; hot water

Some Notes About My Food Journal: So you may take a look at what I ate and think, "Hey, this is the way a diet should work." While you could certainly follow this menu, it's more important to note the big principles in play. There are a couple of things going on here that you should apply to your own eating strategy. You may notice that I generally have the same one or two meals for breakfast every day. It makes my decision automatic so I don't have to worry about what I want (and thus increase the likelihood that I'll over-eat). Pick a few healthy things you like to eat for breakfast—and even for lunch—and make them your go-to choices most of the time. It goes a long way toward removing the chance of impulsive eating that hurts so many people.

I'm just as happy having my scrambled-egg concoction for dinner, or a simple salad, like on Tuesday night. Think simple and redefine what the word *meal* means to you and it'll be easier to stick to good choices.

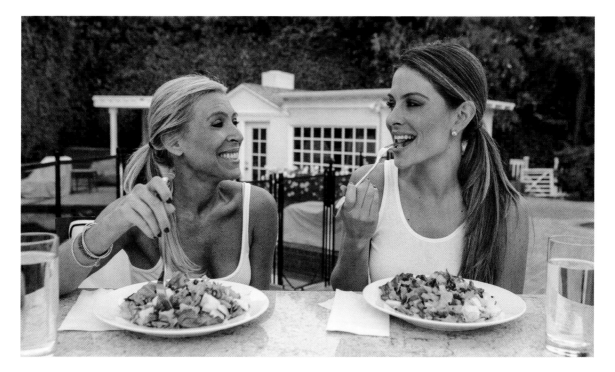

Q What is your philosophy on health?

"Food is thy medicine." Our health is directly reflected upon what we put into our bodies every day, so I really try to choose the most nutritious and nourishing foods that my body needs to stay energized and replenished. I know that taking care of my body now will be the best preventive measure against poor heath as I get older.

Q What's one food people should think of subtracting and one food they should think of adding to their regular diets?

FOOD OPTIONS TO ADD

Garlic - Garlic is a cancer-fighting wonder! The active ingredient in it is allicin, which contains antibacterial, antifungal, antiviral properties known to kill numerous disease-causing bacteria. Try to have one clove a day if possible!

Chia seeds - A wonderful superfood that provides the body with energy and plenty of protein. Chia seeds are a great source of plant-protein, are high in antioxidants and dietary fiber, and also contain eight times more omega-3 fatty acids than salmon!

Coconut oil - Coconut oil can be used for literally everything; it is the superhero of oils. It can be used as a shave gel, lotion, lip balm, hair mask, cooking oil, and delicious dessert addition. The oil's antifungal and antibacterial properties make it a great natural tool for warding off any bacterial or fungal infections. This superfood is easy and inexpensive to consume or use. Simply add a spoonful to just about anything to help reduce inflammation as well as speed up the body's metabolism. I love using coconut oil!

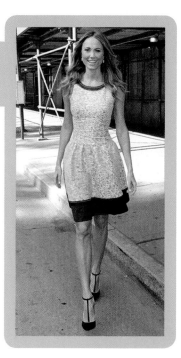

FOOD OPTIONS TO ELIMINATE

I would say that's a toss-up between gluten and dairy. Both can really wreak havoc on the body! Gluten is an extremely common inflammatory allergen that can even cause inflammatory reactions from people without an extreme allergy. As a result, when gluten is eaten regularly, inflammation doesn't become a temporary bodily solution, but something more permanent, which causes the body to become much more vulnerable to other viruses and bacteria. Similarly, dairy is also overconsumed in the U.S, with the average American eating more than 32 pounds of cheese. Our bodies are not built to digest exorbitant amounts of anything. Dairy causes acidosis, which can lead to obesity but also a loss of calcium in the body, resulting in osteoporosis.

Soda - Artificial sugars such as aspartame are incredibly harmful to the body. The sweetener damages and even kills nerve cells by excessive stimulation, which in turn causes several nervous-system-related conditions, including memory loss, Alzheimer's, etc.

Q **What are your favorite healthy snacks, and for when you're on the go?**

My favorite healthy snacks range from my homemade superfood ice creams (no dairy, no gluten, no sugar) to kale chips to pressed juices. I love foods that give me energy throughout the day. I also love a good, quick snack, which is why I generally carry a raw bar like the Elemental Superfood Seedbar with me!

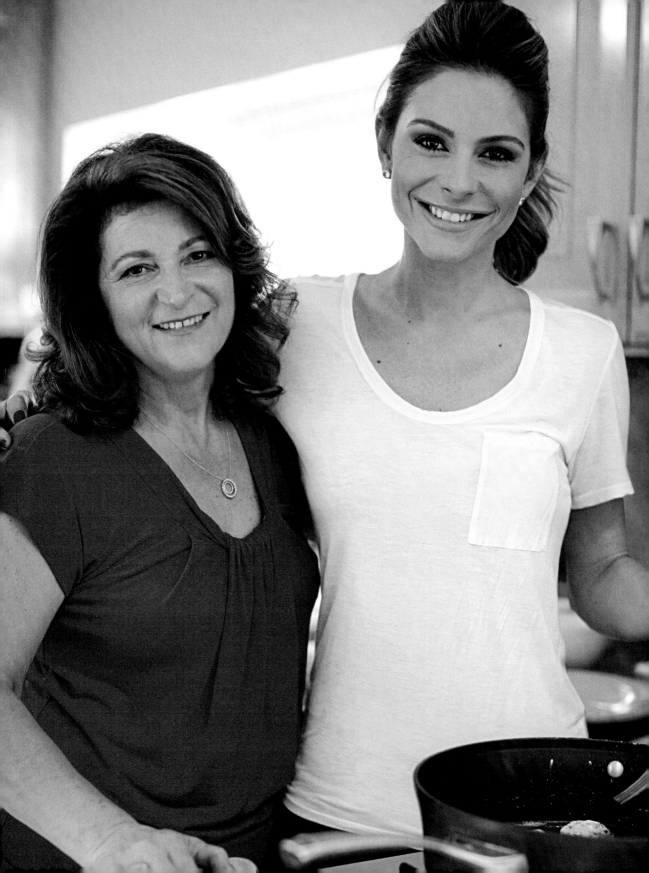

Chapter 8

EveryGirl's Recipes

My mom is a really amazing cook. She learned a lot from my grandfather, who was a chef in Greece. One of the many things that stands out about my mom's cooking is the way she makes vegetables taste so delicious. When I was growing up, we were always eating what was fresh from our garden. Being raised on a diet full of whole and real foods, I gained a deep appreciation for them.

My mom and I spent a lot of time cooking together, and I think that's one of the reasons why I like to cook so much—it brings back so many wonderful memories.

As much as I love to cook, though, I don't have a whole lot of time to spend in the kitchen. Neither did my mom, and most likely, neither do you. That's why the recipes in this chapter aren't just healthy and tasty; they're also really, really easy. These are the recipes I grew up on that my family still eats to this day. They're all vegetarian; you won't find any meat recipes here. Some of the vegetable and grain dishes can be served as a side with meat, poultry, or fish, or they can stand as main courses on their own. I sincerely hope that you enjoy them as much as I do.

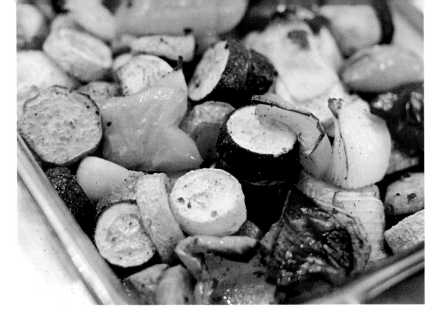

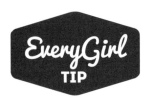

EveryGirl TIP

COOK WITH YOUR KIDS

If you're a parent, know that what you feed your kids today will stay with them for life. Don't think of cooking as just another pressure in your day, but as a way to spend quality time with your family. Even very young children can do some small things to pitch in, such as tearing lettuce leaves for a salad. As your kids get older, you can start giving them simple tasks to help with cooking and use the experience to teach them not just about the "how" but also the "why"—how to cook, how to make healthy foods taste terrific, why healthy foods are healthy for you in the first place. They'll gain an appreciation for whole foods, and that will ensure they go a long way toward thinking of cooking as a way of life and not as a mandatory chore.

Spicy, Crispy, Creamy To-Die-For Roasted Veggies

SERVES 4

2 medium zucchini, sliced into rounds
2 medium summer squash, sliced into rounds
1 large red bell pepper, cut into 8 pieces
1 large green bell pepper, cut into 8 pieces
1 large yellow bell pepper, cut into 8 pieces
1 extra-large onion, cut into large chunks
2 small, thin sweet potatoes, cut into rounds
10 garlic cloves (optional)
½ cup olive oil
Salt and pepper to taste
Crushed red pepper flakes (optional)

Preheat the oven to 450°F.

Combine all the vegetables and the garlic (if included) in a large mixing bowl. Add olive oil and toss the vegetables to coat.

Spread vegetables out on a large baking sheet. Make sure they aren't too crowded; use two baking sheets if necessary.

Bake for 25 minutes, then stir vegetables. (If using two baking sheets, swap their positions so the sheet that was on the bottom rack is now on the top.) Continue cooking another 20 minutes or until vegetables are soft and caramelized. Sprinkle with salt and pepper and crushed red pepper (if included).

The Mouthwatering Special Omelet

SERVES 2

- ¼ cup olive oil
- 1 small onion, chopped
- ½ large yellow bell pepper, cut into strips
- ½ large red bell pepper, cut into strips
- 1 small sweet potato, cut into rounds
- 1 medium white potato, diced
- Salt and pepper to taste
- ½ teaspoon crushed red pepper flakes
- 2 large eggs
- ½ cup crumbled Feta cheese

Heat oil in a large heavy skillet. Add onion and sauté until golden brown, about 3 minutes.

Add peppers, sweet potato, white potato, salt and pepper, and crushed red pepper (if using) and cook, stirring frequently, until the vegetables are tender, about 5 minutes.

In a separate bowl, whisk eggs. Stir in the Feta cheese and pour mixture over the vegetables in the skillet. Cook omelet for 2 minutes, then carefully flip it over and cook until eggs are set, another 1 to 2 minutes.

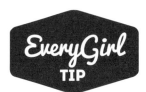

EveryGirl TIP

MY LEFTOVERS TIP

If you do make extra of a dish, serve everyone who is eating a portion and then put the leftovers away *before* you begin to eat. If everything is packed away out of sight in the fridge, you'll be less tempted to load up your plate with that deadly extra serving.

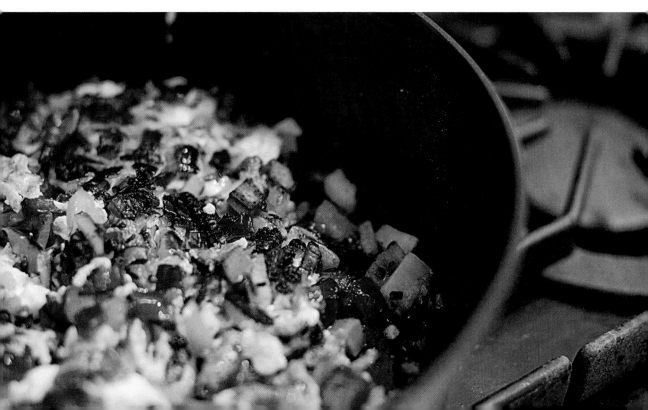

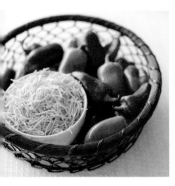

Sweet Stuffed Peppers or "EveryGirl Nachos"

SERVES 4 TO 6 AS AN HORS D'OEUVRE

1   bag of 20 mixed sweet mini peppers (yellow, orange, red)
1   tablespoon olive oil
1   large onion, diced
1   jalapeño pepper, chopped to add taste
1   1-ounce bag of taco mix
1   16-ounce can of refried beans
1   pound of shredded mixed taco cheese

Preheat the broiler.

Line a baking sheet with parchment paper.

Cut each pepper in half the long way. Remove seeds and stem and place pepper halves on the lined baking sheet and set aside.

Heat oil in a medium skillet. When hot, add onion and jalapeño pepper, sauté until onion is golden brown, about 3 minutes. Set aside to cool.

Use a small bowl to mix the taco mix in with the refried beans. Using a spatula or a spoon, fill each pepper halfway with some of the refried beans.

Using your hands, sprinkle the onion and jalapeño mix on top of each filled pepper half.

Sprinkle the cheese evenly over the peppers. Place the baking sheet in the oven about 8 inches away from the broiler and broil until the cheese is melted and golden, 2 to 3 minutes.

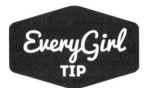

SUNDAY FUNDAY SNACK

We are a big football-watching family. One of the snacks my mom or I will make are my EveryGirl Nachos. Try making them for game day!

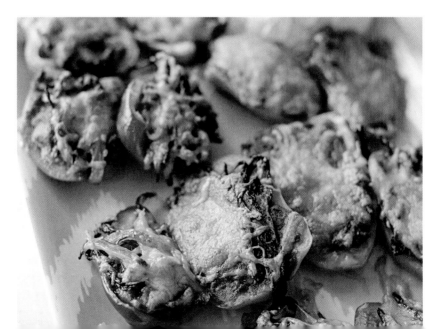

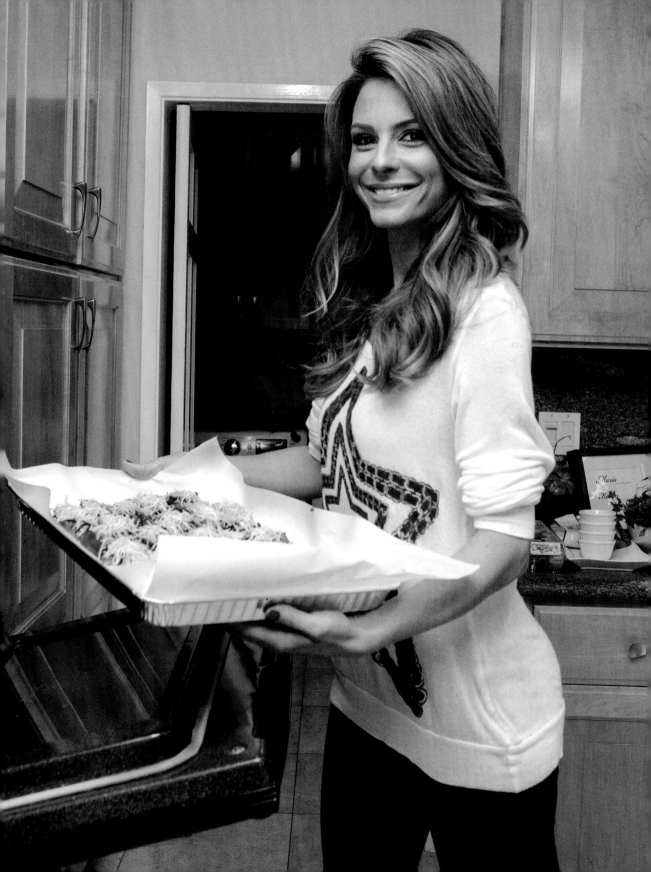

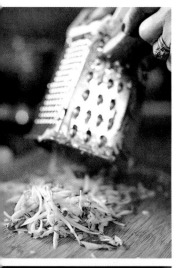

4   large zucchini, grated
½   cup minced Italian parsley
½   cup grated Parmesan cheese
4   garlic cloves, minced
    Crushed red pepper flakes (optional)
1   cup plain bread crumbs
1   large egg
    Salt and pepper to taste
1   cup all-purpose flour
1   cup olive oil (for frying)

Place zucchini in a colander and squeeze out as much water as possible. Transfer to a large bowl.

Add parsley, Parmesan cheese, garlic, crushed red peppers (if using), egg, salt and pepper, and bread crumbs. Mix well.

Form mixture into small balls. Roll a ball in the flour, shake off excess, and place it on a sheet of aluminum foil that you've set out near the stove. Press gently to flatten slightly. Repeat with remaining zucchini balls. Heat the oil in a deep, heavy skillet. Place a few zucchini balls at a time into the hot oil. Make sure not to overcrowd the pan. Fry zucchini balls, flipping them over so that both sides get golden brown. Remove balls with a metal slotted spoon or tongs and place on a plate lined with paper towels to drain. Repeat with remaining zucchini balls.

These are excellent to serve with tzatziki sauce for dipping. (Tzatziki is a yogurt, cucumber, and garlic spread. You can buy it already made at most grocery stores.)

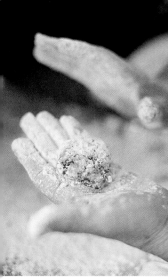

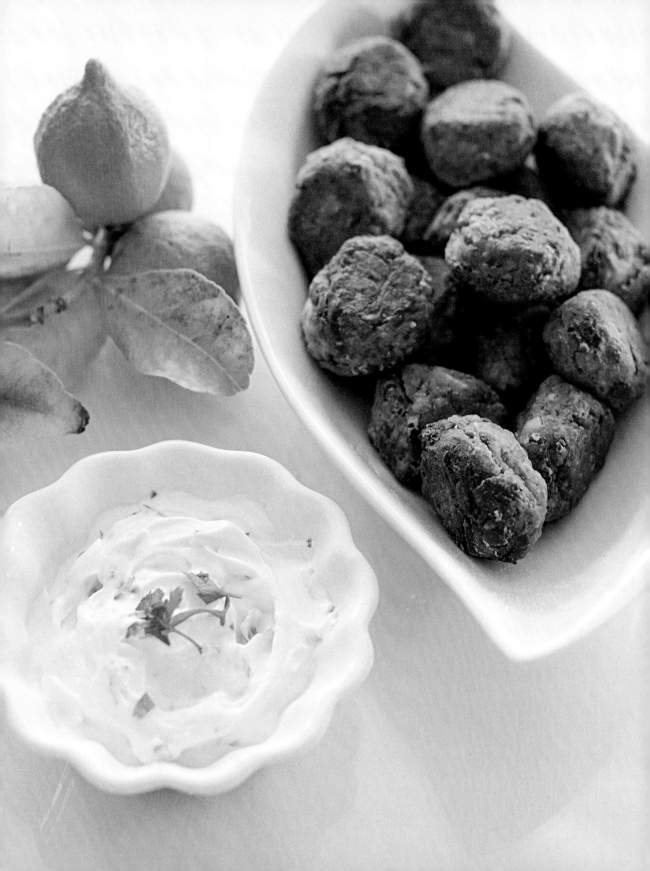

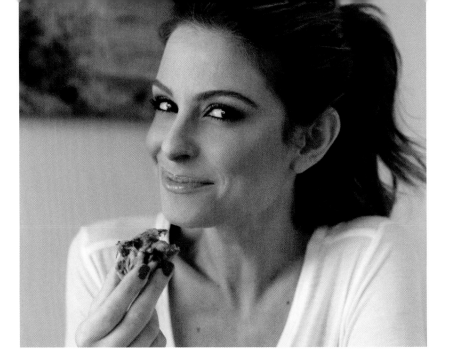

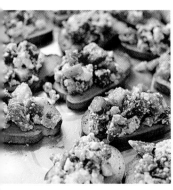

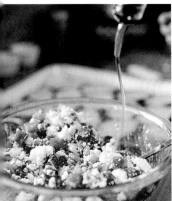

Greek Bruschetta

SERVES 6 TO 8 AS AN HORS D'OEUVRE

1   loaf fresh Italian or French baguette bread cut into 1-inch slices
¼   cup olive oil (for brushing)
4   medium tomatoes, diced
1   tablespoon oregano
    Pepper to taste
1   pound Feta cheese, crumbled

Preheat the oven to 375°F. Place bread slices on a baking sheet and brush each slice with the oil. In a bowl, combine tomatoes, oregano, pepper, and Feta.

Bake bread slices for 8 minutes or until bread is crispy.

Top each slice of bread with some of the mixture.

164

Roasted Sweet Potatoes

3 to 4 medium sweet potatoes
2 tablespoons cinnamon
3 to 4 tablespoons butter, melted (optional)

Preheat the oven to 450°F.

Peel and slice sweet potatoes into rounds about a quarter-inch thick.

Place sweet potatoes sprinkled with cinnamon and butter (if using) in a small baking pan.

Bake for 35 minutes or until potatoes are nice and crispy on the outside and soft on the inside.

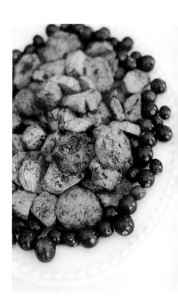

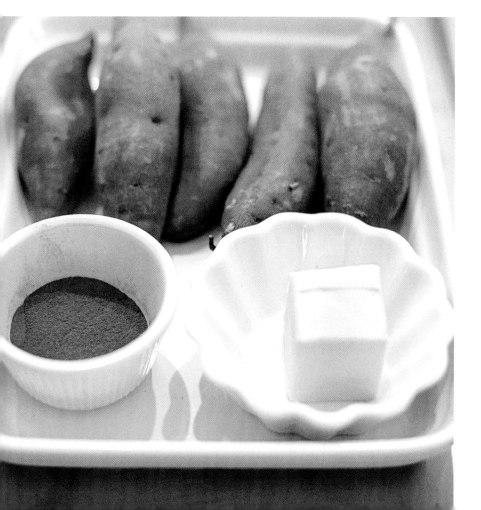

165

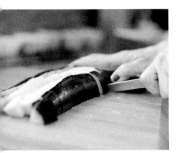

Mixed Baked Veggies

1 medium eggplant, cubed
1 onion, julienned
1 large baked potato, cubed
1 zucchini, cubed
½ cup flat-leaf parsley, minced
3 cloves garlic, minced
 Salt and pepper to taste
½ cup olive oil
4 large tomatoes, diced

Preheat the oven to 375°F.

Combine all of the ingredients in a medium baking pan. Cover the pan with aluminum foil and bake until tender, 35 to 40 minutes.

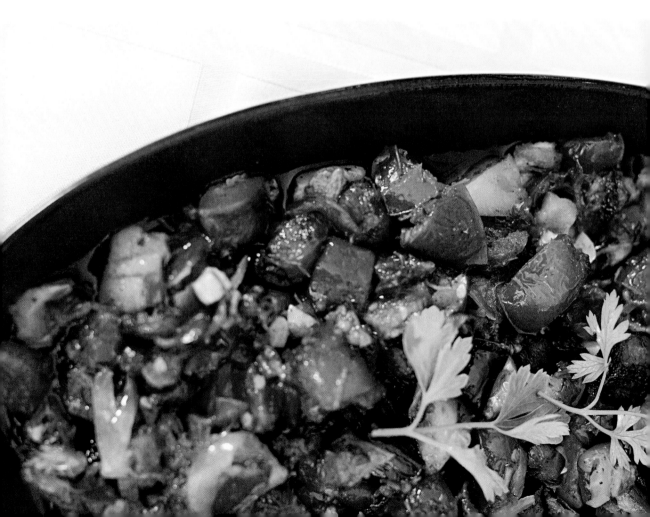

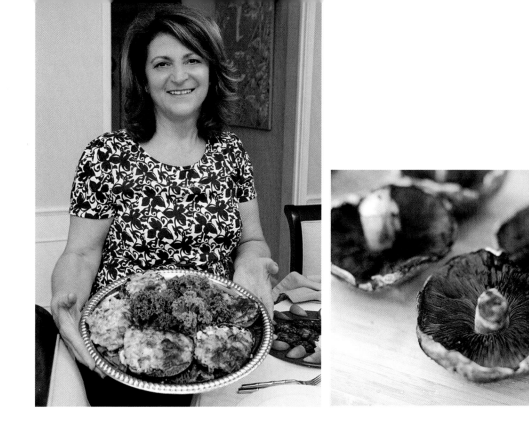

Stuffed Portobello Mushrooms

SERVES 5 TO 6

5 to 6 portobello mushroom caps
1 16-ounce can white beans, drained and rinsed
1 small red onion, chopped
½ red bell pepper, diced
   Salt and pepper
   Crushed hot red pepper (optional)
½ cup Feta cheese, crumbled
1 cup mozzarella cheese, shredded

Preheat the oven to 350°F.

Clean the mushroom caps and place them in a large baking pan.

In a medium bowl, mash the beans gently and mix in onion, bell pepper, salt, pepper, and crushed red pepper. Stuff the mushroom caps with the mixture.

Top with Feta cheese and mozzarella cheese. Bake until the cheese is melted and golden, 15 to 20 minutes.

Tomato Omelet

½   cup olive oil

1   large onion, cut into strips

4   large tomatoes, cut into small pieces

1   jalapeño pepper, minced

    Salt and pepper to taste

½   cup Feta cheese

4   large eggs

Heat oil in a large sauté pan that has a cover.

Place onions on one side of the pan and tomatoes on the other side.

Stir onions and tomatoes separately until the onions are caramelized and most of the water has evaporated from the tomatoes, about 15 minutes. Mix onions and tomatoes together and add jalapeño pepper and the salt and pepper. Cook for 2 to 3 minutes.

In large bowl, mix Feta cheese and eggs. Pour on top of the vegetable mixture, stir, and cover the pan. Cook for 1 to 2 minutes, then flip the omelet over and cook for another 1 to 2 minutes.

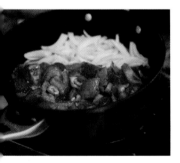

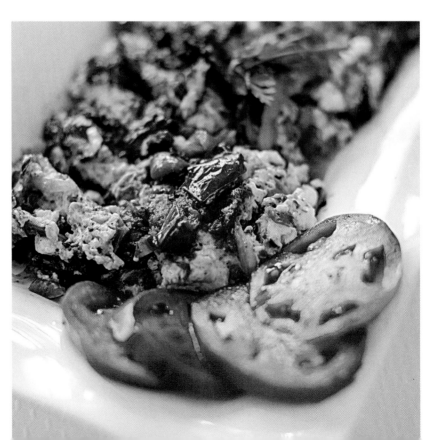

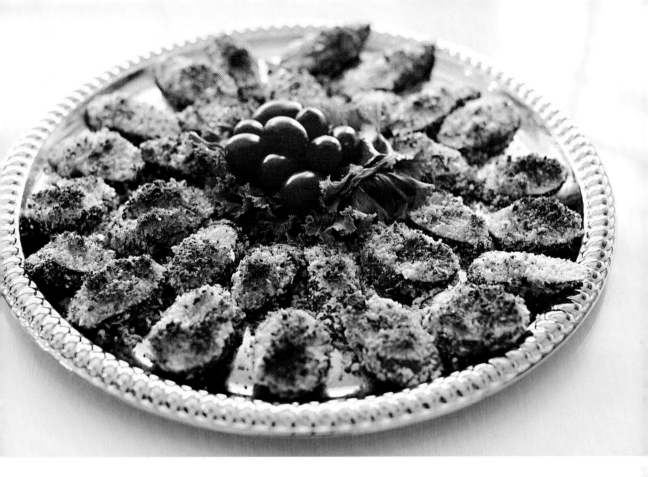

Baked Breaded Zucchini

SERVES 4

1 cup almonds, finely chopped
½ cup Parmesan cheese, grated
1 cup Japanese panko bread crumbs
4 medium zucchini, cut into rounds
3 tablespoons olive oil
Freshly ground black pepper

Preheat the oven to 375°F and grease a baking sheet.

In a large bowl, mix almonds, Parmesan cheese, and bread crumbs.

Brush zucchini rounds with the oil.

Pat each side of the zucchini slices with the almond mixture so that they are entirely coated and place them on the baking sheet. Bake until nice and crispy, about 30 minutes. Sprinkle with pepper to taste.

MARIA'S FAVORITE FOODS

If someone asks me, "What should I eat?" it's hard for me to give an answer. That's because I believe that if you try to follow the 75/25 rule and eat the foods you love, then **that's** what you should eat. So the way I like to answer the question is to change the question: What do **I** eat? You get a sense of my diet in my sample food journal on page 152, but this top ten list will give you a sense of how I put together my meals. There are plenty more that I love (hello, tiropita–Greek cheese pies that are ridiculously out of this world), but these are the ones that I rely on for my tastes and my health.

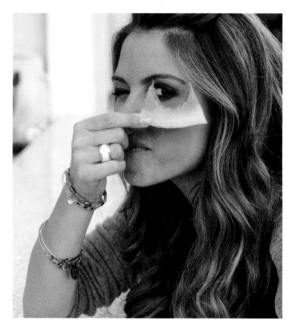

Watermelon: It's my go-to snack for lots of reasons. Besides its sweet taste, watermelon is also a water-rich fruit, meaning that it can help fill you up so that you aren't tempted to gorge later on. Besides being packed with vitamin C, it's also a rich source of the antioxidant lycopene, which has been shown to be a powerful disease-fighter.

Turkey: One of the keys to staying satisfied throughout the day is making sure you get enough protein. Protein keeps you satiated and helps rebuild your muscles after a workout. I like turkey because it's an extremely lean source of protein. It's also easy to include in wraps or salads for lunch or as your main source of protein for dinner.

Eggs: You'll notice in my food journal, I start many mornings with egg whites. That's because I think it's important to get your day going with some protein for both energy and satiety. Even though they're low-calorie, they include both protein and fat to help keep my hunger in check. I also love them because there are so many ways to serve them, such as omelets and scrambled eggs. Wait till you try my mom's egg recipes!

Greek yogurt: *Greek-style yogurt is much thicker than the regular kind; that's because it's strained. So it's a good option because it has less sugar and more protein than other yogurts. Have it with berries, or drizzle on some honey. Try it for a snack, a dessert, or even an on-the-go lunch.*

Lentils: *Love me some lentils. They're filled with protein and fiber, so if you're looking for something to keep you full, you can't beat them. I can put some on a salad or make them part of a wrap or even create a lentil-based soup.*

Feta cheese: *Okay, so you won't typically find cheese on most people's list of diet foods. And there's good reason—cheese is calorie-dense, so having a lot can make your daily calorie counts go off the charts. My Greek roots, of course, mean that crumbly Feta is my favorite, but I also like it because of the strong flavor—you don't need to use a lot. I use it in my morning egg scrambles, but it's also good on salads or in wraps to perk up meat and veggies.*

Kale: *This leafy green is the hot vegetable of our time—and for good reason. It's packed with vitamin C, calcium, and lots of other nutrients. You can use it as a salad base, add it to a wrap, sauté it with garlic and serve it as a side dish, and even sneak it into a smoothie. We all need more vegetables, and I try to include as many as I can, but because of its versatility and health benefits, kale is one leafy green I eat a lot of.*

Almonds: *Packed with healthy fats and protein, almonds are filling and have also been shown to help lower cholesterol and cut your risk of developing heart disease. I keep almonds in my car and in my desk at work. When hunger strikes, I eat a handful, and it tides me over until I can eat a meal. Also fun: Add just a bit of all-natural almond butter to smoothies to give them more substance, taste, and satiating power.*

Potato skins: *Healthy? Nah. But you gotta live it up every once in a while. Of course, real potato skins—not the bar food staple—are quite nutritious. Talk about a good snack: Bake some potatoes and scoop out the middle. Then drizzle on a little olive oil and spices and roast them in the oven. They're delicious and don't have all the calories of the deep-fried version.*

Chocolate chip cookies: *Do not deny yourself chocolate. This is how I like mine delivered. Enough said.*

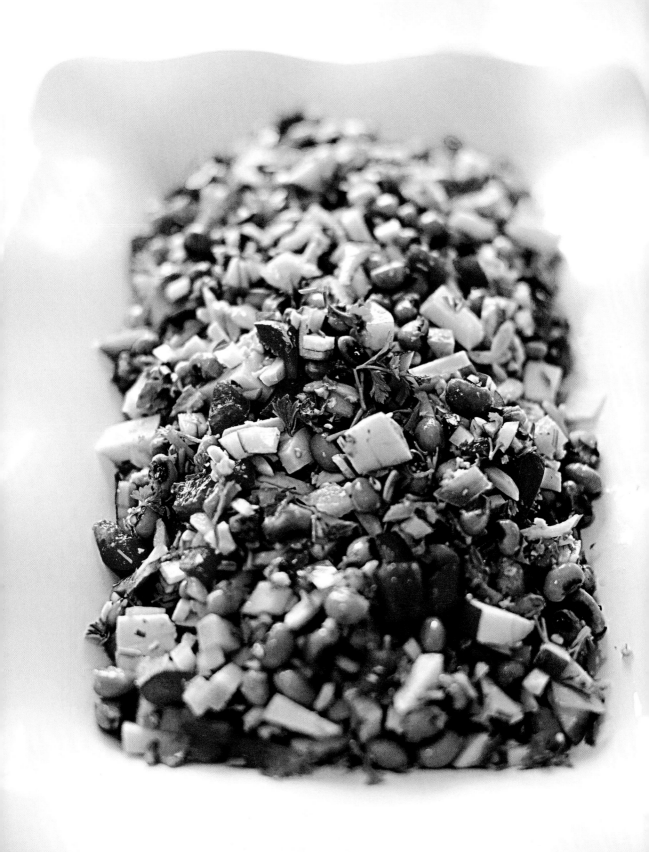

Black-Eyed Pea Salad

SERVES 4

- 1 16-ounce can black-eyed peas, drained and rinsed
- 1 small red onion, diced
- ½ cup of green bell peppers, diced
- ½ cup of red bell peppers, diced
- ½ cup of yellow bell peppers, diced
- 2 tablespoons parsley, minced
- 1 Red Delicious apple, cored and diced
- ½ cup almonds, chopped
- 3 tablespoons olive oil
- 2 tablespoons lemon juice
- 1 teaspoon salt

Mix ingredients in large bowl and serve.

Greek Avocado Delight

SERVES 8 TO 10

- 2 avocados, peeled and pitted
- 8 ounces Feta cheese, cut into small pieces
- 2 garlic cloves
- 2 tablespoons olive oil
- 2 tablespoons lemon juice

In a food processor, mix all of the ingredients. Use as a dip for pita chips, celery, carrots, or other raw vegetables.

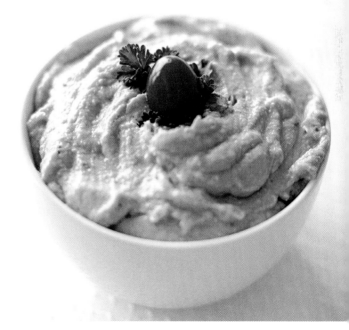

Lentils and Brown Rice

1 cup lentils
3 tablespoons olive oil
1 medium onion, chopped
½ cup brown rice or quinoa, cooked
1 small red bell pepper, chopped
3 tablespoons fresh mint, chopped
3 tablespoons parsley, chopped
Salt and pepper to taste

Prepare the lentils separately by boiling in 4 cups of water until tender, about 20 minutes. Drain.

Heat oil in a sauté pan, add onion, and sauté until caramelized, about 3 minutes.

Add cooked rice and lentils, and stir to combine.

Remove from heat and sprinkle with bell pepper, mint, parsley, and salt and pepper. Serve warm.

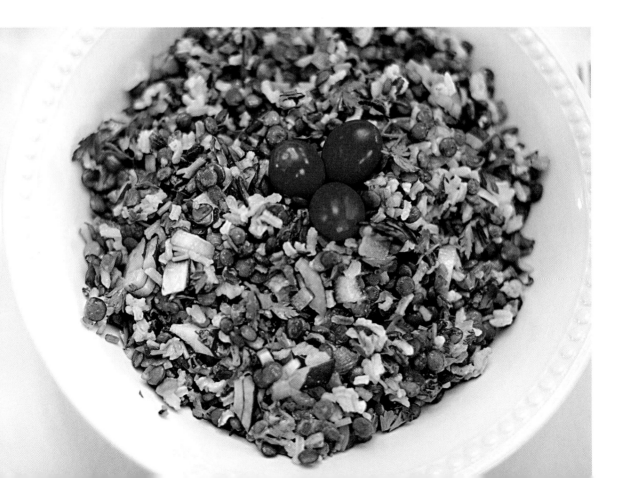

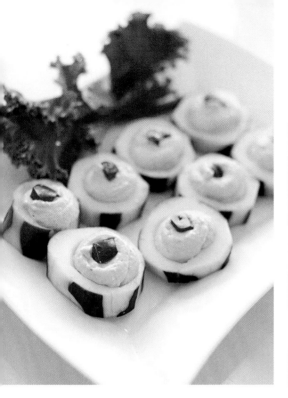

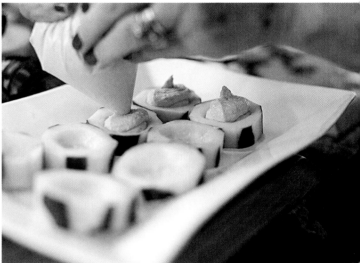

Cucumber Pockets

SERVES 4

2 large European cucumbers, cut into rounds
½ cup hummus
½ red bell pepper, diced in small pieces

Scoop the seeds out of the cucumber with a spoon without cutting the bottom.
You should be left with a small cucumber cup.
Fill each cucumber round with hummus.

Place one piece of diced pepper on top of each for decoration.

Eggplant Veggie Falafels

2 large eggplants
1 cup plain bread crumbs
½ cup almonds, finely chopped
½ cup all-purpose flour
½ cup fresh mint, chopped
2 cloves of garlic, minced
1 large egg
1 cup fresh parsley, minced
  Salt and pepper
1 cup olive oil (for frying)

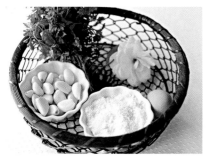

Preheat the oven to 365°F.

Place whole eggplants on a baking pan and bake until cooked, 15 to 20 minutes. In a medium bowl, mix together breadcrumbs, almonds, and flour.

When eggplant is cool enough to handle, place it in a food processor and blend for 30 seconds.

Add mint, garlic, egg, parsley, and salt and pepper to the food processor and blend for 30 seconds.

Use a large spoon to scoop out a spoonful of the mixture and form into a ball. Dip the ball into the almond mixture to coat. Place on a sheet of aluminum foil. Repeat until you've used all the mixture.

Heat the oil in a deep, heavy skillet.

Place a few eggplant balls at a time into the hot oil. Make sure not to overcrowd the pan. Fry eggplant balls, flipping them over so that both sides get golden brown. Remove balls with a metal slotted spoon or tongs and place on a plate lined with paper towels to drain. Repeat with remaining eggplant balls.

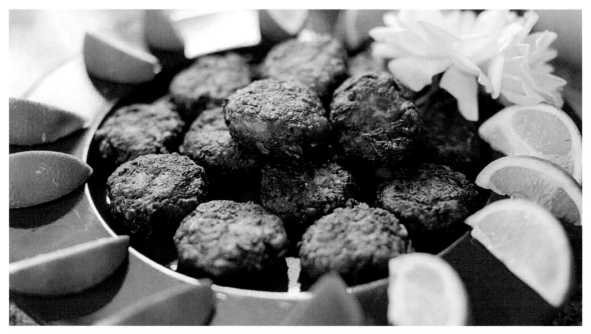

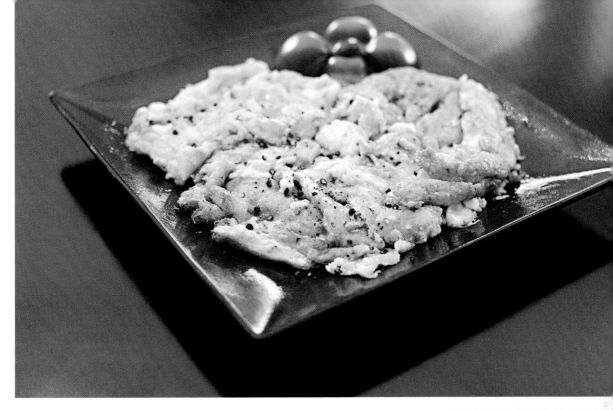

Greek Egg Omelet

SERVES 1

3 tablespoons olive oil
2 large eggs
½ cup Feta cheese, crumbled
1 teaspoon black pepper
1 teaspoon crushed red pepper

Heat oil in a deep skillet.

In a medium bowl, mix eggs, Feta cheese, black pepper, and crushed red pepper.

Pour mixture into the skillet. Cook until bottom is set, about 1 minute. Do not stir. Flip omelet over and cook for another 1 to 2 minutes.

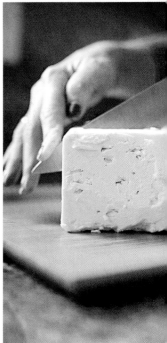

Papou's Baked Potatoes
& Eggplant Casserole

½ cup olive oil

1 small onion, diced

2 large onions, julienned

5 garlic cloves, minced

1 cup fresh parsley, minced

2 bay leaves

Salt and pepper

1 7-ounce can tomato sauce

2 large eggplants, sliced into $1/8$-inch slices

2 large white potatoes, sliced into $1/8$-inch rounds

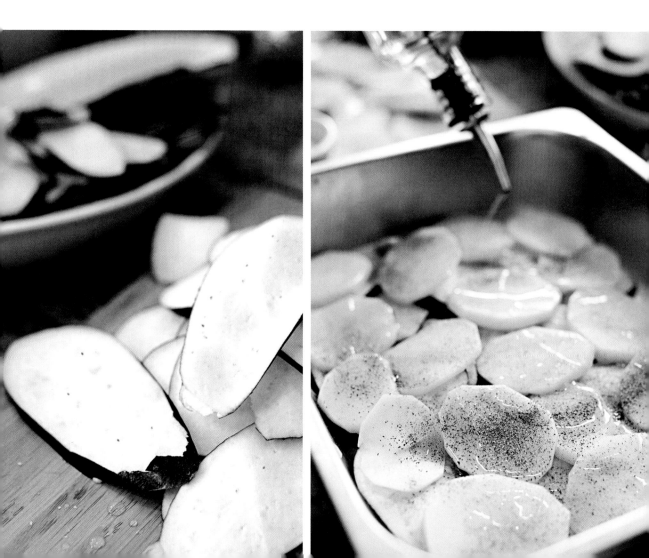

Preheat the oven to 350°F. Heat oil in a large skillet. Add diced onion and sauté until caramelized, about 3 minutes.

Add julienned onions, garlic, parsley, bay leaves, and salt and pepper and sauté until tender, 3 to 5 minutes.

Add tomato sauce. Cook until sauce is warmed through, 1 to 2 minutes. Remove bay leaves and set onion mixture aside.

Oil the bottom of a deep baking dish. Cover the bottom with slices of eggplant and potatoes, overlapping the slices. Top with half of the onion mixture.

Layer with remaining eggplant and potatoes. Cover with the other half of the mixture.

Bake for about 35 minutes until golden brown.

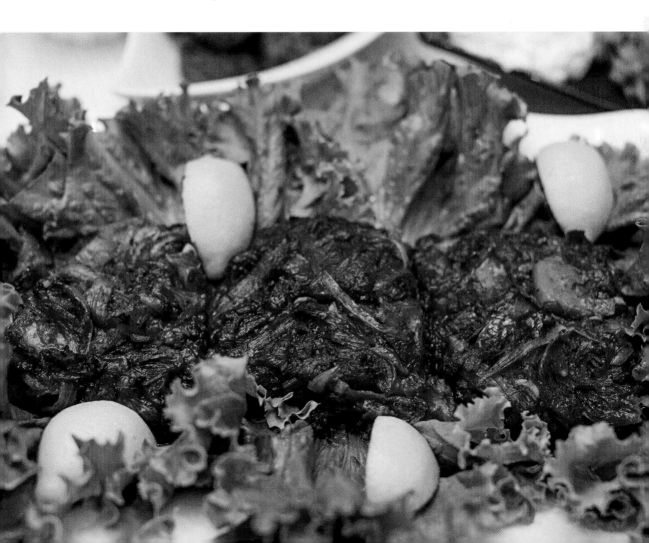

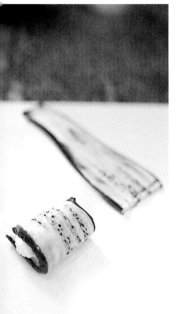

Stuffed Eggplant with Feta and Ricotta Cheese

2 large eggplants, sliced lengthwise into ½-inch strips
¼ cup olive oil (for brushing)
½ pound Feta cheese, crumbled
1 cup ricotta cheese
1 large egg
Black pepper
1 teaspoon crushed red pepper
1 16-ounce jar marinara sauce

Preheat the oven to 375°F.

Grease a pizza pan with some of the oil and place the eggplant slices on the pan. Brush the eggplant slices on both sides with the oil and bake until soft, about 15 minutes. In a large bowl, mix Feta cheese, ricotta cheese, egg, black pepper, and crushed red pepper. Remove eggplant from the oven and let cool. Leave the oven on. When eggplant is cool enough to handle, spread each slice with the cheese mixture. Roll each slice and place them seam-side down into a baking dish. Pour the marinara sauce on top of the eggplant and bake 20 minutes.

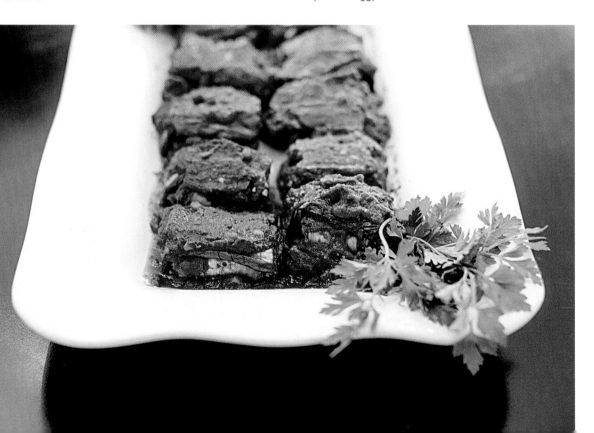

Quinoa-Stuffed Zucchini

4 large zucchini
1 cup quinoa, cooked
1 medium red onion, diced
1 cup red and green bell pepper, diced
3 tablespoons olive oil
2 tablespoons fresh mint, minced
2 tablespoons fresh parsley, minced
2 cloves garlic, minced
1 cup crumbled Feta cheese

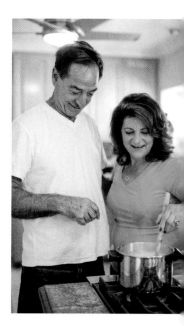

Preheat the oven to 350°F.

Slice the zucchini in half lengthwise, and then again widthwise. Scoop out the insides and place them skin-side down on a baking sheet.

In a large bowl, mix quinoa with onion, bell peppers, olive oil, mint, parsley, and garlic.

Fill zucchini halves with mixture. Sprinkle Feta evenly on top.

Bake for 35 minutes.

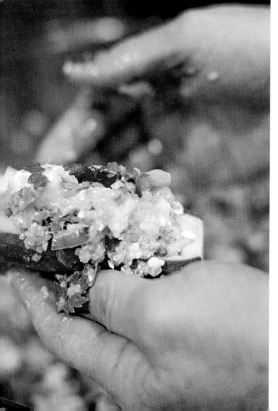

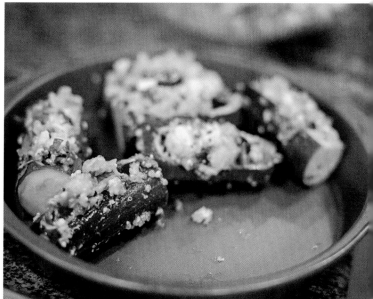

Orzo Salad

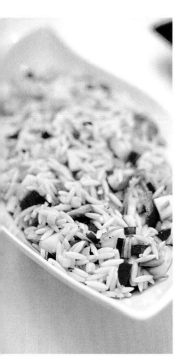

1 cup orzo
½ yellow bell pepper, minced
½ green bell pepper, minced
½ red bell pepper, minced
1 cup cucumber, chopped
3 tablespoons fresh parsley, chopped
1 small red onion, diced
1 cup Feta cheese, crumbled
½ cup frozen corn kernels, defrosted
½ cup carrot, shredded

DRESSING:

½ cup olive oil
¼ cup lemon juice or vinegar
1 clove garlic, crushed
Salt and pepper to taste

Cook orzo according to package directions until just past al dente. Drain orzo and rinse in cool water. Drain again.

In a large bowl, combine orzo with the rest of the ingredients.

To make the dressing, whisk the dressing ingredients together.

Pour the dressing over the orzo salad and mix gently. Serve at room temperature. You can also refrigerate and serve cold, but don't pour the dressing on until ready to serve.

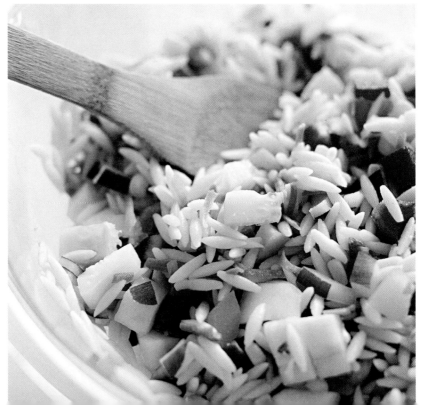

MARIA'S KITCHEN ESSENTIALS

Besides the usual pots and pans, here are the things I recommend you have in your cooking arsenal so that preparing healthy food is both easy and fun.

Two plastic cutting boards, one for meat/fish and one for fruit/vegetables.

A Magic Bullet blender for protein shakes, salad dressings, and more.

A measurement conversion chart for quick reference when making recipes (and to help you with portion control).

An instant-read thermometer to help you cook meat and poultry to perfection.

A salad spinner to help dry your lettuce—wet lettuce doesn't hold the dressing. You can also use the spinner to dry fresh herbs.

An 8-inch chef's knife. You can do almost everything with it, and it makes prepping vegetables a breeze. Go to the store and try out a few. It should be sturdy, sharp, and feel comfortable in your hand. Chef's knives tend to be pricey, but you can find a very good one for under fifty dollars.

2 pairs of tongs, one long handled and one short handled.

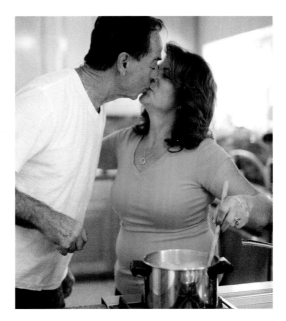

Lots of plastic containers in different sizes, which make it easy for you to prepare and store food a few days ahead of time. If you've got something healthy in the fridge that just needs to be warmed up, you're less likely to resort to takeout. And if you can make your own delicious lunch to take to work, you won't be as tempted to grab whatever is available when you're starving.

A Microplane zester for use on citrus fruits and also to grate cheese or chocolate finely.

An electric kettle to heat your water.

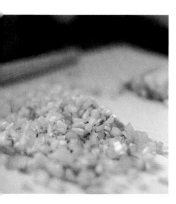

Maria's Favorite Tuna Fish

1 12-ounce can white water-packed tuna
½ cup celery, minced
½ cup plain bread crumbs
  Salt and pepper
¾ cup low-fat mayonnaise
3 teaspoons crushed red pepper

Mix all ingredients well and serve on top of salad or on sandwich bread.

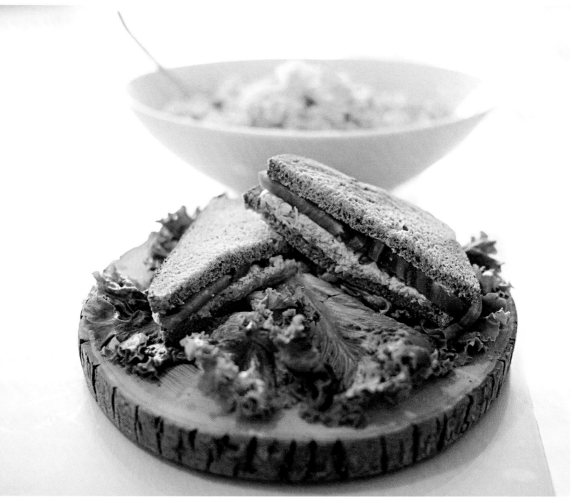

Yogurt Mélange

SERVES 1

4 ounces nonfat Greek yogurt
1 tablespoon walnuts, crushed
1 tablespoon golden raisins
¼ cup fresh blueberries or other berries
1 tablespoon honey
1 tablespoon fat-free whipped topping

Mix yogurt with walnuts, raisins, and blueberries.

Transfer to a serving bowl. Drizzle with honey and top with whipped topping.

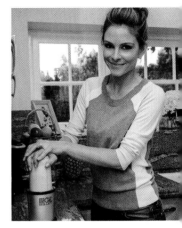

MY FAVORITE SMOOTHIE

Harley Pasternak's Apple-Nut Smoothie. It's nutritious, delicious, and filling—doesn't get much better than that. I started his shake plan while getting ready for a cover shoot and stuck with it. His shakes are delicious and have everything you need in them. I love this shake because I can run around in the a.m. and get all my work done and not be tied to my desk eating breakfast.

5 raw almonds
1 red apple, unpeeled
1 small frozen banana, chopped
¾ cup (6 oz.) nonfat plain Greek yogurt
½ cup nonfat milk
½ teaspoon ground cinnamon, or to taste

In a blender, finely grind the almonds. Add in the remaining ingredients and blend. Add in water or ice cubes if you prefer a thinner smoothie.

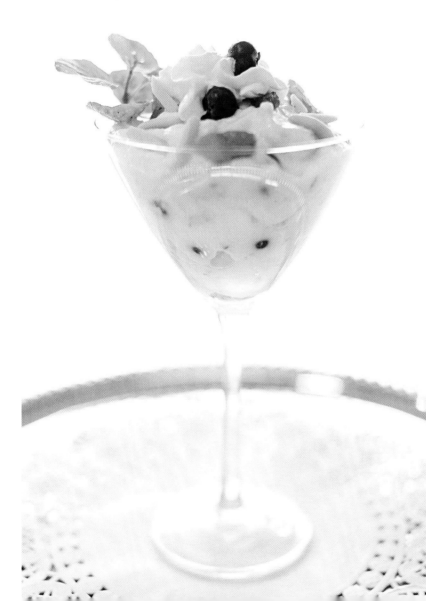

185

Maria's Mediterranean Delights

I'm so excited to announce my new line of frozen foods called Maria's Mediterranean Delights. The dishes were inspired by the amazing dishes my mother and grandfather, who was a chef, made. The same recipes I grew up eating. They are wonderful Mediterranean dishes that are both healthy and delicious.

I've partnered with the Parthenis family, owners of Grecian Delight Foods, and together, we're making Greek and Mediterranean food accessible to all. We're sourcing all-natural ingredients, some of which are imported from Greece and throughout the Mediterranean. If you've never tried Greek delicacies such as moussaka, pastishio, spanakopita, dolmades, and the sweet-tasting baklava, you're in for a treat (and even if you have tried them, these frozen foods will be a wonderful, low-maintenance way to have these dishes more often). Though they're not fat-free (there's nothing wrong with a little fat), they are made with all-natural products and are preservative-free.

Check it out at *mariasmediterraneandelights.com* or call (800) 621-4387 for info on where to find it.

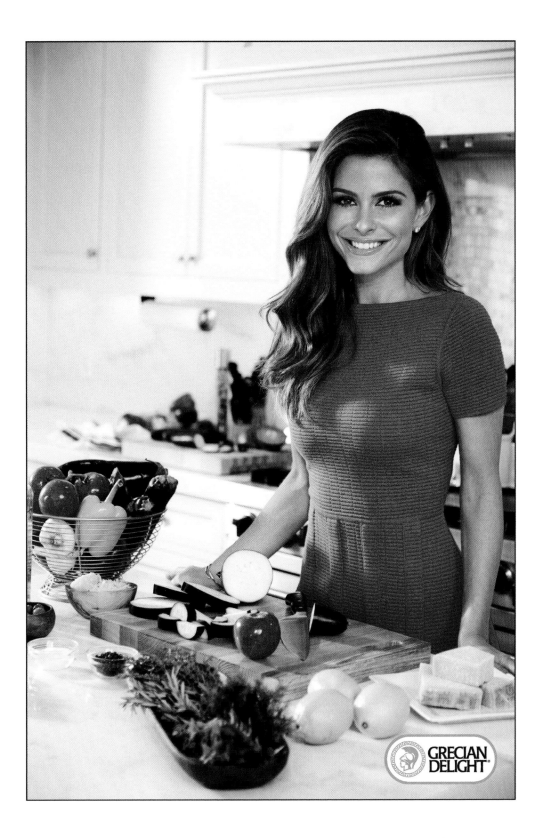

What is your philosophy on weight loss?

I'm not pro-diet, but I am pro-portion control. It's not about losing weight, it's about being healthy and happy!

What are your favorite pre- and post-workout foods?

Since I have a hectic schedule, I almost always work out in the early morning—my workout being yoga. So I usually wait until after to eat. My meals really fluctuate with the weather, so if it's chilly, a warm bowl of oatmeal (no dairy!) or brown rice with olive oil. If it's hot out, a nice smoothie or some juicy grapefruit with a little agave. And an Americano, of course!

What's one food people should remove from their diets and one food they should add?

Sodas, ditch them! Everyone's body is different, so it's hard to name one thing that everyone should add. Water doesn't really count, but most people need to hydrate more. That being said, I'll say arugula!

What are your favorite healthy snacks?

Almonds! I love raw almonds and always have some in my bag for a quick pick-me-up. A nice, crisp Fuji apple with a little almond butter is also delish.

What do you grab to eat or drink during your day when you're tired?

A smoothie or juice is perfect for a quick boost. My fave is spinach, apple, lemon, ginger!

When you need to prep for a photo shoot or the red carpet, what do you do beforehand?

I usually will stick to fresh juices and have one meal a day.

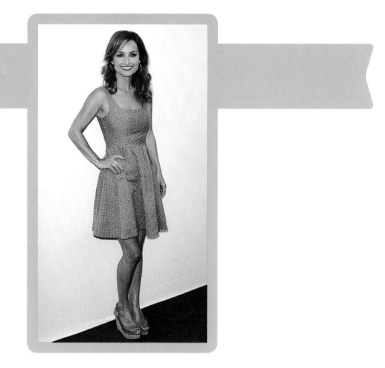

Q **What's your advice for watching what you eat when eating out?**

Try to order appetizer courses (I order two apps instead of a main course), or I order a main course and have them box up half! Also, dressing on the side!

Q **What does a typical day look like food-wise for you?**

Oatmeal (made with water) with olive oil and salt for breakfast, a piece of fruit for a snack, a nice green salad and protein for lunch, afternoon snack is iced Americano and sometimes a piece of toast with almond butter and sliced strawberries, and dinner is whatever the fam is having. Usually a small meal!

Q **What body image issues do you share with the EveryGirl?**

Due to the nature of my job in front of the camera, I have a lot of moments where I look in the monitor and don't like what I see for one reason or another. It's a daily opportunity to catch myself and be kind and say nice things instead of the comments we are brought up to say and that are based on unrealistic expectations. I really believe to look your best, start with love.

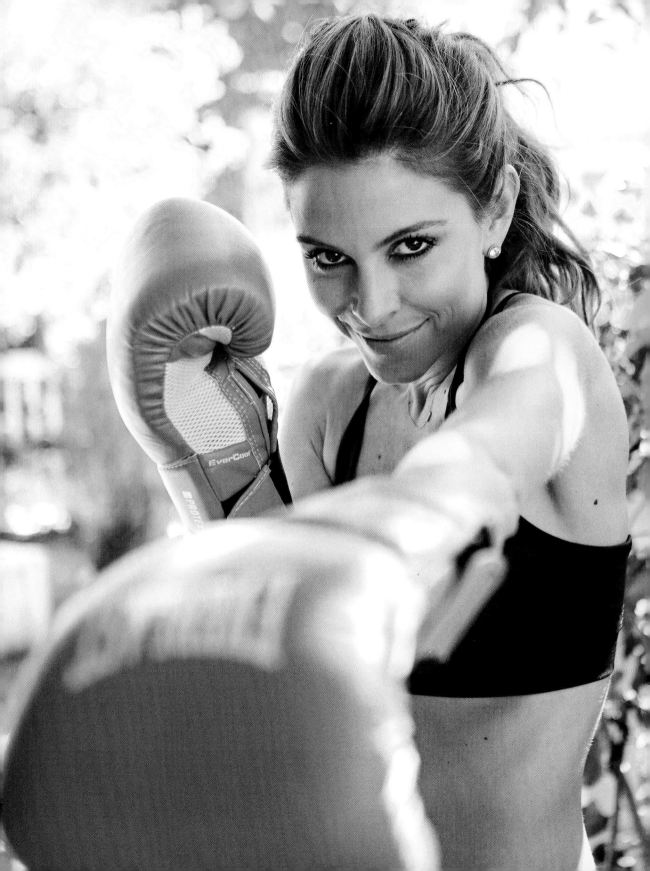

PART THREE

EveryGirl

FITNESS

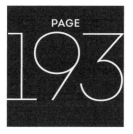
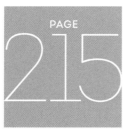
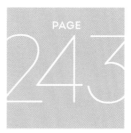
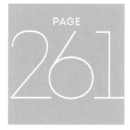

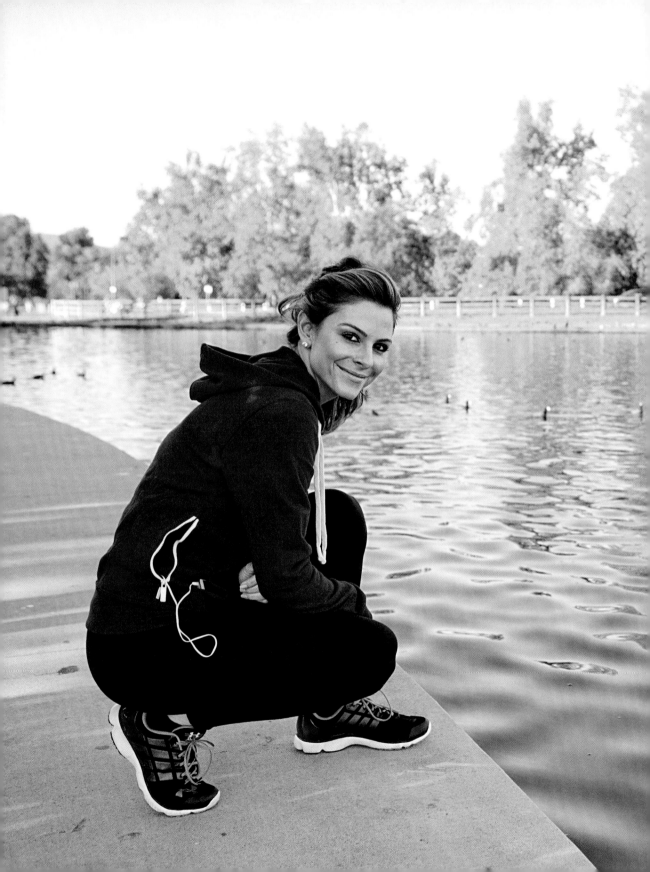

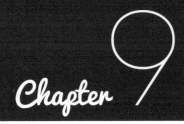

EveryGirl's Approach to Fitness

I've always been a sports fan. Growing up, I loved watching the Boston Bruins, the New England Patriots, and WWE Pro Wrestling with my father. Along with playing basketball, these were some of my fondest childhood memories. But I didn't get interested in working out until I was about thirteen.

After I begged, pleaded, and cried, my extremely strict Greek father agreed to let me participate in the Miss Perfect Teen beauty pageant. When Harry Bouras—the manager of the Channel, a nightclub in Boston that my parents cleaned—caught wind, he scored me an appointment with this amazing photographer named Jean Renard, who was also supermodel Niki Taylor's manager at the time. Jean Renard told me that at 5'7½", I was a little short to model. However, if I wanted to make a go of it, I should begin working out with a trainer to tone up. And so I started meeting with trainer Ina Krueger two or three times a week. It was tough for two reasons:

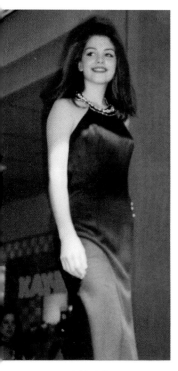

↑ Modelling in a *Seventeen* magazine fashion show in Boston. I was 15 years old.

I had to travel into Boston for the workouts, and Ina trained me like I was a bodybuilder! It was hard, heavy lifting, but I learned the basics of working out and firmed up all over. Still, I couldn't afford the sessions or the long commute, so I eventually gave up. (No time, no money . . . sound familiar?)

Later, I joined a gym in my hometown of Medford, Massachusetts, and worked out on my own on and off through high school and in college at our school gym. It didn't make much of a difference, though. No matter how hard I tried, I couldn't keep the weight off. Back then I was under the misconception that exercise alone could help you lose weight. I assumed that I could eat whatever I wanted and work it all off at the gym. And when that didn't work, I got discouraged. As a result, I never could find my workout rhythm.

After I gained all that weight in college and then made a conscious long-term decision to get in shape, I got back into the exercise groove. My cousin Anthony, who was a mentor to me growing up, went to high school with Debbie Maida, a local athlete and soccer star. Debbie was also training people on the side and Anthony, the smart and generous person that he is, hired her to train me for one session. Debbie created a basic workout plan for me that I used for nearly a decade. She taught me that I didn't need a celebrity trainer and I didn't need anyone to guide me three times a week, either. All it took was a single hundred-dollar session with Debbie to get everything I needed—the rest was up to me.

Debbie's plan included jump-

← The Original EveryGirl Workout (Debbie's). See it in action on page 297

194 THE EVERYGIRL'S GUIDE TO DIET AND FITNESS

ing rope, push-ups, sit-ups, and some strength-training moves I could do with light dumbbells. I'd get my cardio (short for cardio-vascular exercise, which I'll address later) on the elliptical machine. I hit my local gym, five minutes from my house, three to five days a week, but I struggled at first. Debbie wanted me to do forty-five minutes on the elliptical, and the first week I could barely do five minutes. Eventually, I ever so gradually built up to forty-five minutes, but it took a good deal of time.

Since that session with Debbie, I've tried all kinds of exercise routines. Sometimes, I do structured workouts, sometimes I play basketball for hours at a stretch, and other times, I'll just run up stairs for a few minutes when I have time or pedal while I work at my FitDesk. You don't need to do a crazy workout every time you exercise. As I've said before, the most important thing is that you move throughout the day. Move, move, move. Like the great Jack LaLanne said, there's enough exercise in just avoiding being inactive. If you keep moving throughout your day, you'll burn calories, stoke your metabolism, have more energy, be less likely to overeat, be more productive in life, sleep better, have fewer health problems—I could go on and on. Before I outline some of my favorite workouts, I want to share my major fitness principles. It won't be a surprise that my philosophy on exercise is similar to the one I have on eating well: There are a number of good ways to do it, but you don't have to be super-rigid about the process. Find what works best for you and what you enjoy most so that you'll continue to do it.

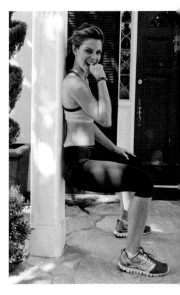

ABE: Always Be Exercising

By now you're probably saying to yourself, "I get it, Maria! I need to be active and keep moving throughout my day." While that's true, I want you to take that mentality to the next level. I want you to Always Be Exercising as well: continually seeking and creating

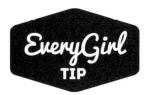

Don't engage in long, strenuous workouts right out of the gate. Chances are you'll end up too sore and tired to continue long-term. Just like with change to your diet, start slowly and increase gradually.

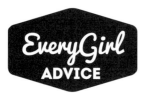

Think of exercising throughout your day as a means to get out of going to the gym. That's what I do!

exercises within your daily activities and routines. I'm constantly looking for new ways to squeeze in a workout as I go about my day. For example, I never sit on toilets. (This may be oversharing, but stay with me.) I hover over the seat. It's like doing a squat, and it tones your thighs and butt. Trainers always say you should hold your last squat for as long as you can, and this is basically the same principle. It's a small thing, but when you do stuff like that over the course of a day, it adds up.

While I'm standing and waiting for a ride, I'll stand on my tiptoes repeatedly to build my calf muscles. Carrying plastic bundles with handles to and from my car, I'll do biceps and triceps curls. I have friends who use one liter water bottles to do biceps curls and shoulder presses as they talk on the phone. Another friend uses play time with her baby to exercise. She does squats and sit-ups while holding and playing with her. During the day, be conscious and creative in your daily tasks, turning them into calorie-burning, muscle-building opportunities whether you're carrying the laundry upstairs or lugging a bag of dog food to your car.

It's all about trying to move as much as you can. Again, don't look for the convenient way to get things done, look for the *active* way to get things done. I opt to walk instead of drive and take the

"To break out of a plateau, keep challenging your body in new ways. That can mean going harder or longer with your workouts. Intervals or sprints will help you burn more calories in less time."

—Betty Wong, editor-in-chief, *Fitness* magazine

stairs instead of the escalator. And when I take the stairs, I try my best to run them and to feel that extra burn in my quads. It honestly does keep me toned, and it proves that you don't always have to do X workout at Y time with Z frequency. It's just as effective to live a life in which you incorporate activity anywhere and anytime you can. Sure, sometimes, that means you'll do a formal workout, but sometimes you'll just walk around the block or to your errands or speed walk to the bathroom or water cooler instead of sauntering. It means you'll take stairs instead of elevators. It means vacuuming, mopping, or polishing at a pace that resembles an actual workout.

Exercising Isn't an Excuse to Eat More

There will be times after a taxing workout that you'll want to eat more. It's okay to do so occasionally, but don't have the mind-set that you *can* or *need* to eat more because you're exercising. Most workouts burn far fewer calories than you think. Eating more because you're working out is more likely to just lead to extra calories and those extra calories will only negate the work that you've just done. Remember that the bulk of weight loss is a result of eating fewer calories, not exercising more.

Weight Loss Mainly Comes from Eating Less, but . . .

Changing my diet is mostly what helped me lose weight, and research does show that it's hard to lose weight through exercise alone. Still, working out helps immensely. When you exercise regularly, you feel healthier and more confident. Psychologically, you tend to want to avoid bad foods and to eat well. You have more energy, too, which may be crucial, since weight loss can drain energy.

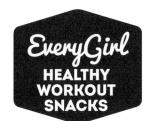

EveryGirl HEALTHY WORKOUT SNACKS

Be armed with healthy post-workout snacks to help stave off hunger. A glass of skim milk works in a pinch, but I've provided some more substantial options below. They've got a combination of carbs and protein, which helps you refuel and repairs muscle.

Nonfat Greek yogurt with fruit

Banana and almond butter (I spread it right on the banana)

Low-fat chocolate milk

Tuna on whole-wheat bread

Turkey breast and hummus on whole-wheat bread

Hummus and pita

Turkey and cheese with apple slices

Turkey breast and hummus roll-ups

Turkey breast and mustard roll-ups

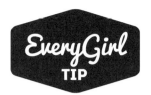

EveryGirl
TIP

Invest in a hands-free headset for your phone. It may not be attractive, but it keeps your hands free to do other things like exercising. I use my headset while I'm power-walking or using resistance bands.

Working Out Becomes More Important After Weight Loss

After you've lost weight and have established healthier eating habits, exercise becomes more valuable, which is why I encourage you to begin incorporating exercise into your routine in Phase Two. Once the weight is lost, this is when it's time to build some muscle and endurance. When I say muscle, I don't mean bulk or ripped muscle—though if that's your preference, go for it. I mean getting toned and strengthening your core, arms, and legs so that you stay strong and productive for many years to come. Plus, experts say that exercise really is the thing that separates people who gain the weight back from people who don't.

Set Goals, but Have Realistic Expectations

Whether it's walking ten thousand steps a day, which is my current goal, or jogging three times a week to prepare for a marathon, fitness goals inspire and motivate you to keep a consistent training program. The problem is, just as goals are sometimes with dieting, people often set fitness targets that are far out of their reach—at least at first—and in that way they're not set up for success.

EveryGirl
TIP

CONSIDER WORKING OUT AT LUNCH

I do this often. It's a good way to avoid eating poorly midday. Plus, you get your day's exercise out of the way and over with.

If Eating Less *and* Exercising More Is Too Much . . .

At some point I want you to exercise. It helps prevent depression and, again, will keep you more independent, confident, energetic, mobile, strong, and healthy for the next fifty years. But if working out *and* changing your diet is overwhelming, then *don't do it*! Just focus on the diet end of things and ramp up the activity in your day. Have a sense of urgency in the things you do, always be moving, and resist convenience.

"Do anything . . . do something. It's better than nothing. Just get in and swim five laps. Just run once around the reservoir or just bike for 20 minutes. ANYTHING is better than nothing, and if I start I usually keep going and do more than I had planned or bargained for."

–Lucy Danziger, editor in chief, *Self* magazine

Do What You Can When You Can

My schedule changes every week—sometimes every day, every hour. So I can't lock into a routine too much. As you can guess by now, I do what I can when I can. Sometimes I do yoga on my front lawn before I hop in my car to go to work, sometimes I'll run up the stairs on breaks, and other times I'll get to the gym for an official workout. Whether it's a 10-minute stretch session, a walk around the block, or some pushups at your desk, if your busy schedule prevents you from having a set workout plan, then just do what you can when you can.

Half a Workout Is Better Than Nothing

I have friends who have this fitness philosophy: If they can't get their entire planned workout in—say, a three-mile run—they figure, why bother. I have a different outlook. Go for a mile run instead. There are days when Kev is headed out to the gym, but I stop him because I need him on a conference call or to talk to him about

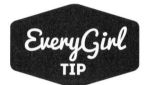

YOU DON'T NEED AN HOUR TO TRAIN

Those days are gone! Harley Pasternak taught me that you can get an effective workout in just twenty minutes (or less). Interesting how ninety-five-year-old Jack LaLanne said the same thing in one of his final televised interviews!

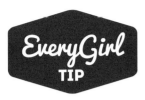

EveryGirl TIP

BABY WIPE SHOWER

If you're worried about having the time to work out and shower and get back to your desk, do what I do. I carry baby wipes to give myself a quick "shower" and deodorant and perfume to refresh.

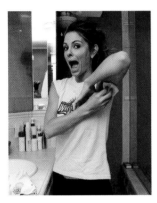

→ My friend and trainer to the stars Andrea Orbeck. Love her—she always keeps it fun and different! We work together when I have to shoot a cover for or something like *Self* magazine a few years ago. We'll set a goal for around 5 sessions.

something. When that happens, he grabs the resistance bands, dumbbells, or the barbell we keep under our bed, and he'll use them for a smaller workout while we discuss whatever we have to discuss.

If your day gets crazy and you can't do a full workout it's okay to do a smaller one. Maybe it's working with some resistance bands at your desk or in front of the TV, or only half the time at your gym. Bottom line: Something is better than nothing.

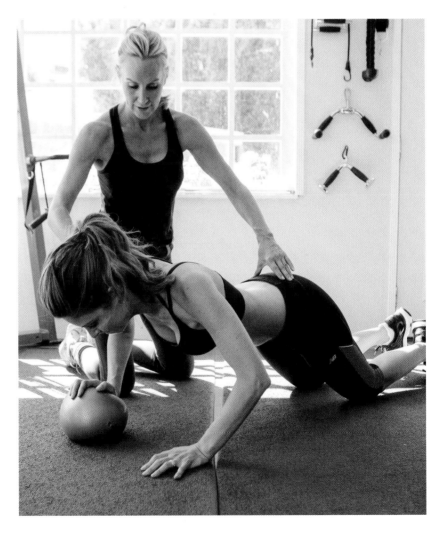

THE EVERYGIRL'S GUIDE TO DIET AND FITNESS

Make This One Investment Up Front

Learn some basics from someone who knows. Just like I did when I started, hire a trainer for just one session. It's worth the investment to learn some basics from a professional. You don't have to be locked into an expensive regimen for weeks, months, or years (though obviously, if you find it helpful and have the means to do so, then go for it). Be honest with him or her about what you want to get out of that workout: a written plan tailored to whatever your specific goals are—to lose weight, build muscle, tone up, run a race, or a combination of things. If you have a gym membership, a trainer usually will show you how to use the machines and free weights and give you a routine to adhere to for free. A good trainer can teach you how to get a good workout with inexpensive equipment—like resistance bands, an exercise ball, and a mat—or no equipment at all. In fact, you can get an excellent workout just using your body weight for resistance. Regardless, just get something on paper, then stick to it as best you can. Think of what you learn from that workout as a recipe—you can add more of this, use less of that, putting in different moves in different combinations. As long as you're keeping good form and not putting yourself at risk of injury, you can concoct any variety of combinations to keep your workouts fresh and fun.

Don't Let a Trainer Hurt You

I recall doing a segment for a show with this one trainer who was pushing me beyond my limits. I knew that I was straining my hamstring and wanted to let up, but she kept pushing me. I was younger then, and the segment was on camera, so I obeyed her. I ended up doing some major damage to my hamstring that troubles me to this day. You know your body better than anyone. If a trainer pushes you too hard to the point of injury, make sure you ignore them and stop.

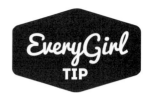

WHEN EXERCISING— ALWAYS BE MOVING!

I have never understood how people can spend more time at the gym yapping and walking around than they do actually working out. You'll do more for your body and your schedule if you stay focused. Just like you should always be moving and have a sense of urgency as you go about your day, you want to do the same at the gym or wherever you work out as well. Don't rest between exercises. Jack LaLanne didn't, and neither should you! On your break from triceps kickbacks, do your biceps curls. Alternate your back exercises with your chest exercises. This workout style is called supersetting. You work opposing muscle groups one move after another. It's faster and it's more intense, enabling you to burn more calories. If you don't want to do this, do jumping jacks or jump rope between sets. Don't just stand there!

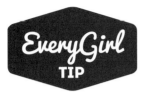

**MAKE THE MALL
YOUR TRACK**

When the weather
prevents you from walking
or jogging outdoors hit the
local mall. Malls are
veritable tracks where you
can walk briskly and get
many steps or even miles in.
Many malls open early just
to accommodate walkers.

Take Advantage of Your Surroundings

Is there is a park or a gym near where you work? Before we moved to Universal, we shot *Extra* from a venue called the Grove, an up-scale outdoor shopping mall of sorts. Across the street was a park—the perfect place to squeeze in a workout, weather permitting. I got my co-host, Renee Bargh, to split the cost of a trainer with me, and for forty dollars, he gave us both an awesome forty-minute workout. It was convenient for after work or on our lunch breaks.

Make Workouts Convenient

I had to travel quite a way to get to the first gym I joined, and I eventually ended up quitting. It's hard enough to get motivated to go to the gym to begin with; you don't need anything else stopping you. If you want to work out in a gym, find one that's as close to home or work as possible. If you're going to work out at home, then all the better. You can exercise before you go to work or after. Convenience really makes a difference.

↓ Selfie with friends on
our girls' hiking day!

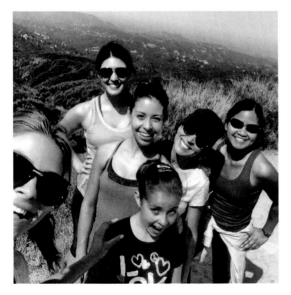

Team Up

I love to work out with friends. It's a great way to catch up, and it helps keep you motivated. If you want to work out with a trainer, it can even save you some money because you can split the cost. My friend Rachel and I do this all the time. You can't beat the incentive. When I was on *Dancing with the Stars*, one of the things that kept me motivated throughout was not wanting to disappoint Derek. And that's a major reason why teaming up works: You don't want to let your partner down by not

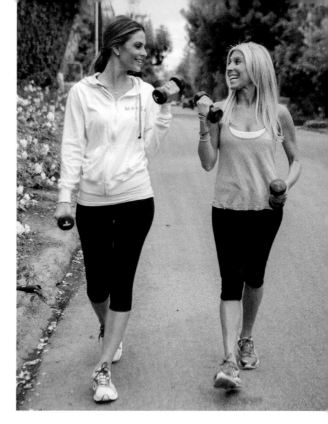

showing up for your run, training session, or Saturday hike. Find a friend, a family member, a coworker with similar goals and similar abilities and see if you can start some kind of routine. Maybe you meet once a week at first and over time increase the sessions. Pretty soon, you'll have created a connection through fitness that keeps you moving—and reaching your goals. When I schedule basketball games with friends I'm less likely to bail, because I don't want to disappoint friends who are looking forward to the game.

Have a Meeting?
Do It Over a Hike!

I have had some of the most insightful breakthroughs in business and in life when walking or hiking with Kev, Rachel, or other friends and coworkers. Next time you have a meeting, whether it's to figure out some business matter, to plan a vacation or an event, or even to settle a family squabble, try working things out while you walk. Do you really think that sitting across from someone at a meeting table would be better? Walking and hiking is so much more relaxed and less official; it tends to yield much better results. Plus you get an amazing and healthy workout in to boot.

Find What Works for You

I'm all about saving money—I already told you how I had doubts when Keven wanted to buy the Bowflex a decade ago. I was sure it would be used for a month or two and then become a dust

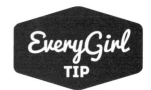

FOR MOMS:
MAKE THE MALL
YOUR STROLLER RINK
I see a lot of moms do this in groups. They attach a small boom box to one stroller then, in unison, push their babies around the mall at a brisk pace. It's a great way to team up, get fit, and beat the cold.

HOW I BEAT MY ASTHMA WITH EXERCISE

Anyone who's had asthma knows the panicked feeling of not getting enough air. Many people describe an asthma attack as trying to suck in oxygen through a straw. Trust me, I've seen many hospitals due to attacks. While asthma is sometimes caused by allergies or colds, some people have what's called exercise-induced asthma—the tubes that carry air to your lungs narrow during exercise and make it hard to breathe. But what's really interesting about all of this? The problem can also be part of the solution. I was able to beat my asthma completely while I was dancing and training on Dancing with the Stars.

Keven was always concerned about how often I had to use my steroid inhaler. Even though doctors say the steroid level in the inhalers is safe, he would always look at me and say, "But, Maria, it's still steroids. What toll will this have on you long-term?" I didn't know the answer, but I also believe that chemicals we put into our bodies can have some kind of negative effect. The problem was that it was literally the only way I could breathe at the time—until I began my dance training on Dancing with the Stars, *that is.*

At first, rehearsals were like doing slow workouts. We would have to perfect the routine and the steps. We were always moving, but it was sort of a gradual cardiovascular workout. As a result, my lungs never got inflamed enough to need the inhaler. Over time, Derek and I built up to faster steps,

and guess what? I still didn't need the inhaler. In the past, I would run fast on the treadmill and my lungs would get inflamed and I would need my inhaler. Because I built up slowly over time, my asthma and my need for the inhaler waned. I later learned from Dr. Michael Roizen, chief wellness officer at the Cleveland Clinic, that frequent, but gradual exercise can actually calm the respiratory system and eliminate exercise-induced asthma altogether. If you build up your endurance and lungs slowly, you can probably do the same.

The experience has motivated me to focus on maintaining my fitness level more than ever—because I never want to use that inhaler again! While certainly some diseases and conditions need advanced medical attention or medication, it's yet another example of how diet and fitness can mend your health.

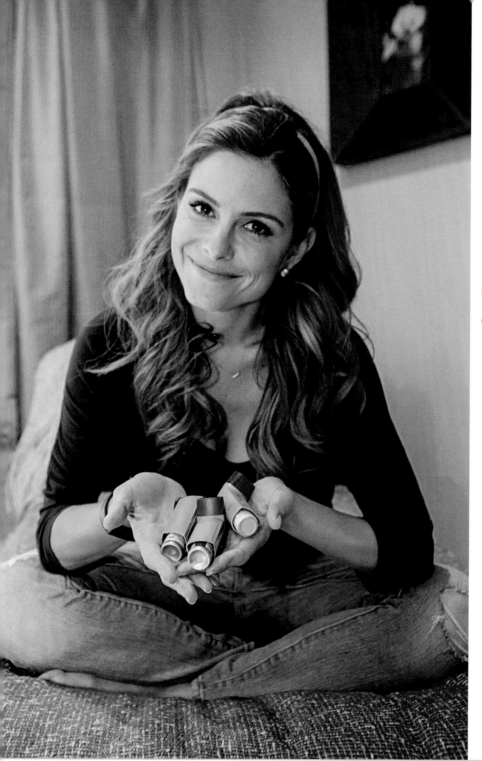

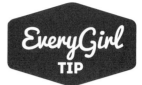

INVEST IN HEPA AIR FILTERS

Jessica Alba recommends adding Hepa air filters to your heat or A/C unit. I just added them to my home. I not only see less dust, but I'm breathing better, too. The filters cost under one hundred dollars. You can also buy portable, electric air filters if you just want one for your apartment or bedroom.

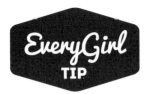

WORK OUT IN KAIZEN!
Whether the workout is a
success or not, remain in
kaizen. Always be open to
new exercises, workouts, and
techniques. I'm constantly
changing mine.

collector, but Kev proved us all wrong by using it for many years and getting great results. Just like with dieting, whatever gym, tool, or workout plan works for you, then do it! I don't care if you use a Jane Fonda workout video from the 1980s! If that's what you like and that's what's going to motivate you to exercise, then I'm behind you 100 percent.

Often trainers or other experts will insist that certain exercises or equipment are the very best. But if *you* don't feel that they are yielding the desired results, they won't do you any good. Like diets, what works for their bodies or their client's bodies may not work for your body. If something doesn't feel right or you're not getting the results you want, you're likely to quit, so change things up until you find what's right for you.

And Keep Looking If You Need to!

Tastes and interests may change, and workouts and equipment may need to be switched up. Remember how Kev got bored after ten years of using the same equipment? We all need new inspirations to keep going. I certainly do. Investing in new equipment for our home gym remotivated him. Don't be afraid to switch out workouts, gyms, or equipment. Finding the right program takes trial and error, you may find a number of workouts you really love, and alternate between them.

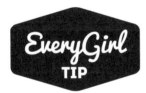

**ALTERNATE WORKOUT
ROUTINES**
Jack LaLanne and other
experts recommend
changing up workout
routines as often as
every 30 days.
Change is proven effective
for muscle development

It's Not About Sculpting Muscles, It's About Building Your Core

Toning your body and getting trim are the by-product. The real value is the amazing endurance, energy, and mobility you gain when you exercise properly. That means working on your core muscles—the ones deep inside your abdomen and back—and not just the ones

206

THE CELLULITE FIX

Nobody wants cellulite, but many women, even thin women, do have it. Cellulite isn't different from any other kind of fat, and exercise will help you minimize it or even get rid of it.

The reason women get that orange-peel appearance is because the tissue connecting our fat cells has a honeycomb structure. Think of overfilling one of those mesh shopping bags with something soft and squishy. Whatever you put in the bag is going to punch out through the holes. It's the same idea on your body. When skin is thin, it is more noticeable.

Men don't tend to get cellulite because their connective tissue has a different structure, and they have thicker skin. Genes play a role and so does aging, because as you get older, skin loses some of its elasticity.

Unfortunately, there aren't any across-the-board surefire fixes; strengthening the muscles in the dimpled area can help smooth your appearance, and simply losing some fat can have a similar effect. For me, eating lighter and cleaner—not having any of my indulgence foods for a week—seems to reduce the appearance of cellulite sharply.

When I was on the road covering the 2008 campaign trail, I got addicted to chips. Soon I saw cellulite creep onto my thighs. But as soon as I cut the chips, the cellulite went away. Ladies, it IS possible!

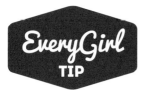

EveryGirl TIP

WORKING OUT LEADS TO BREAKTHROUGHS OF ALL KINDS

Whether you're having problems with friends and family or weighing tough business decisions or feeling stunted creatively on projects, working out may just get you the answers you need. It's happened for me many times. A good workout gives me a solution—it just comes to me. Having that time to yourself, when your mind is focusing only on simple exercises, provides you with peace and puts you in a frame of mind to truly think and see things clearly. It's like meditation, but you're burning calories at the same time.

everyone sees, like your abs or your arms. Strong core muscles help you in your day-to-day activities. Sitting up straight in bed without using your arms, squatting to pick something up off the ground or carrying heavy bundles are all easier when you have a strong core. Those of you in your twenties who played sports in high school or have natural muscle tone may take this all for granted. But once you hit thirty, even if you were a former jock, if you're not exercising or investing in fitness, you'll lose more and more core mobility, strength, and endurance. Remember, as women on the fifty-year plan we all need to be as energetic, active, independent, and strong into our seventies and beyond. Building your core is the best way to ensure that.

↗ I keep these bad boys in my trunk for emergency Rollerblade dates!

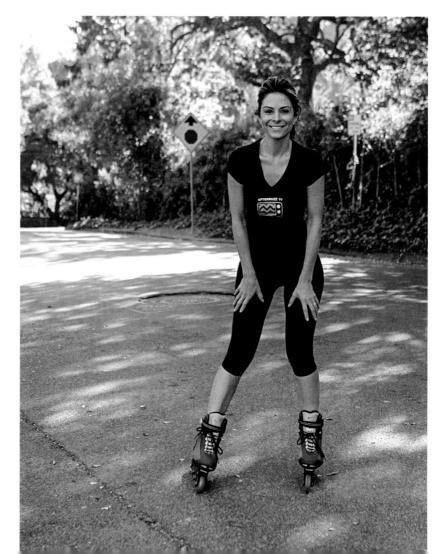

TANNING

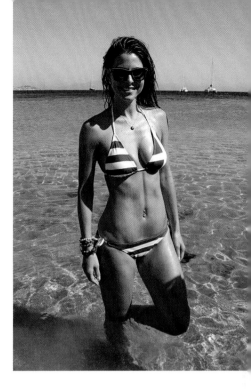

I used to hate being pale, but lately, I've learned to embrace my fair skin. I know that many light-skinned women do like being golden or tan because it makes your whole body look slimmer. Self-tanners are good options for many people (apply them at night), or try a spray tan at a salon. Either way, you get good results without the danger that comes from the sun or a tanning bed, which I don't recommend.

These are the steps I take if I'm going to the spray-tan booth to make sure I get an even glow:

1 Lotion your hands and feet with barrier cream, then dry off thoroughly with a towel. This hydrates your hands and feet to avoid streaking.

2 After wiping, re-apply barrier cream to the soles of your feet and the palms of your hands. Tan palms are a dead giveaway!

3 Be sure to rotate your body while being spray-tanned, so inner thighs and sides get treated, too.

4 Hold five seconds after the spraying is done.

5 Exit the booth and wipe the barrier cream off your palms and soles with a fresh towel.

6 Quickly towel-dry your face and then dry off your body with another clean towel.

7 Get dressed.

8 Use baby wipes to clean your soles and palms only. This will reduce or eliminate orange coloring.

9 Lather your hands and feet completely with lotion and then wipe them dry up to your ankles and wrists.

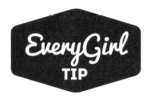

PUMP UP

When I'm going sleeveless or wearing a short dress at big events like the Oscars or the Emmys, I'll do a few quick exercises just before or after I get dressed. I'll do calf raises using a set of stairs and use resistance bands to work my arms. I don't work up a sweat, but I do give my muscles a jolt, and that tightens them up and gives me that sculpted look for the evening. Do the same before your big events or nights out.

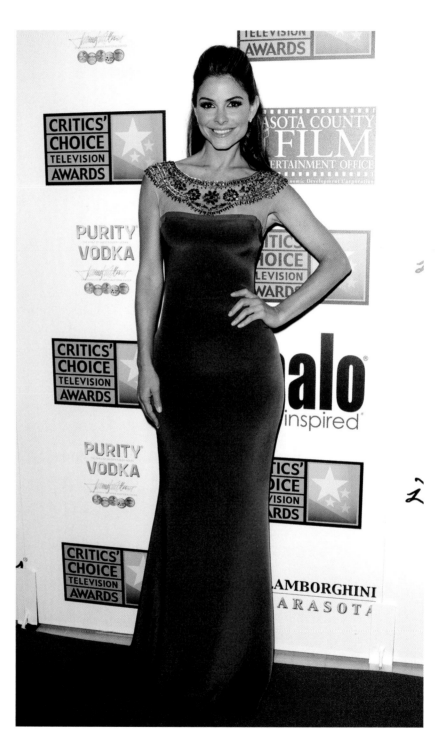

↗ On the red carpet wearing Marchesa for the Critics' Choice Television Awards.

THE EVERYGIRL'S GUIDE TO DIET AND FITNESS

TRACK YOUR STEPS

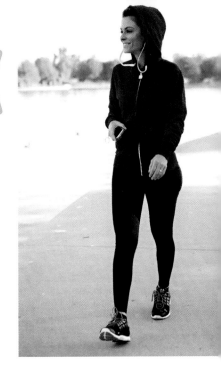

Remember when I talked about my goal to walk ten thousand steps a day? I use my Fitbit, a little gadget that I wear on my wrist to make sure I get them in. The Fitbit measures how many steps I take and how many calories I burn as I go about my day. It's very motivating—I'm always trying to see if I can burn a little more, take a few more steps, and constantly stay in motion. I recommend this or a pedometer to help you track your movement. Here's what a recent week looked like for me. I generally get my 10,000+ per day.

DAY →	1	2	3	4	5	6	7
CALORIES BURNED	2,098	1,958	2,307	2,093	1,999	2,328	2,270
STEPS	8,272	7,208	11,333	9,832	6,713	13,836	13,586
DISTANCE	3.71 MILES	3.21 MILES	5.02 MILES	4.36 MILES	2.97 MILES	6.13 MILES	6.02 MILES

A WEEKLY TOTAL

What my Fitbit told me I did for one week recently:

TOTAL STEPS	TOTAL DISTANCE	TOTAL CALORIES BURNED	WEIGHT CHANGE	AVERAGE TIME TO FALL ASLEEP
70,780	31.42 MILES	15,053	0	3 MINUTES

What are some of your mantras for staying motivated?

Don't cheat yourself; treat yourself (in moderation). :) Every time I am on the stairs, I tell myself, just five more minutes! That keeps me distracted for a little bit and then before I know it I have done more than five minutes. LOL.

What is your best advice for someone struggling to lose weight?

You can't lose in a day! It takes time. Stay focused and don't get discouraged!

What are your favorite healthy snacks?

LOVE hummus. I eat pretzel crisps or Wheat Thins with it. I also love apples and raw almonds. All of these are perfect for being on the go. When I am craving something sweet, I will drink a diet Snapple.

How do you stay in shape?

I work out regularly. I try to stay on working out five days a week. You have to have your mind, body, and soul all in the right light. It's not about a number; it's more about my personal goal and determination.

Favorite body part/least favorite....

The best parts of my body are my booty and my legs! I hate my arms!!

What is your biggest struggle diet-and-fitness-wise?

Fitness actually isn't a struggle for me. I love to work out! My problem is that I am such a foodie. With such a big family, there are always treats and food around. I am best friends with food, so I just treat myself to the things I like in moderation.

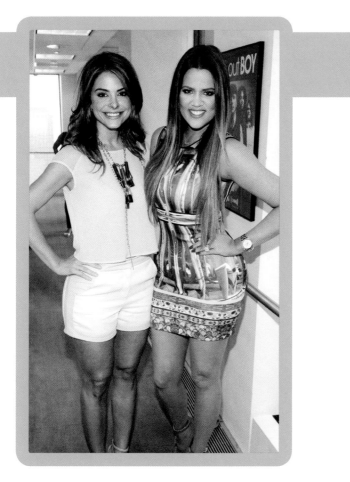

Q **How do you deal with guilt when you've eaten something not in line with your goals?**

I will work out harder the next day. I will make myself do extra cardio and then that makes me not want to repeat what I did. LOL. But I also try not to beat myself up too bad about it because it's okay to love food and enjoy it! Just like I said, take it all in with moderation and you are good to go!

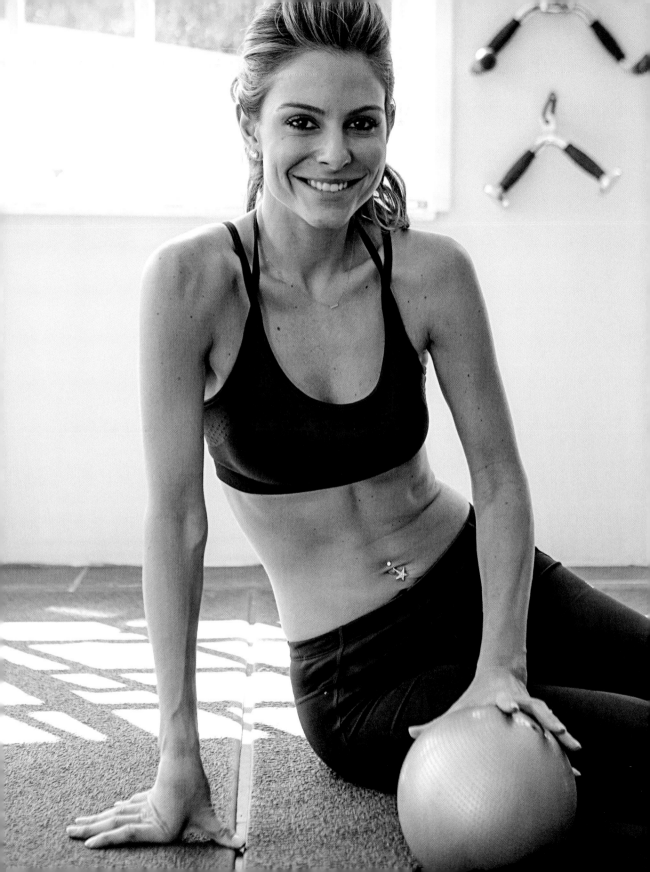

Chapter 10

EveryGirl's Guide to Gyms and Exercise

The best workout routine is truly the one that works for *you*. If it doesn't fit your life and you don't like it, you aren't going to do it. That's why this chapter is about giving you many ideas and options in the hopes one or more of them will suit you. Feel free to mix and match. I just want you to move, sweat, and enjoy how you feel when you're exercising. And I promise, the more you embrace the fun and the amazing feeling a good workout can give you, the more apt you'll be to continue and the better chance you'll have of getting the lean, energized, and healthy body you want.

The Basics

Before we dive into specifics, it's important—especially if you're fairly new to exercising—to get a grasp on the different kinds of workouts there are. They all have advantages. Any type of exercise will burn calories. Some exercises are certainly more intense than others and burn more calories, but how effective they are also depends on how intensely you're working. The categories:

AEROBIC/CARDIOVASCULAR (CARDIO) EXERCISE: This is any exercise that raises your heart rate for a steady amount of time. Examples are running, swimming, cycling, rowing, cross-country skiing, using an elliptical machine, dancing, climbing stairs, and walking fast. Cardio is great for your heart health and will also burn plenty of calories depending on the time you spend doing it.

HIGH-INTENSITY INTERVAL TRAINING (HIIT): So what happens when you take your cardio exercise and instead of going at the same rate and pace for a certain period of time, you change up the intensity—go fast for a few minutes, then slow down for a few minutes, and repeat and repeat and repeat? That's high-intensity interval training. This kind of activity will fry some serious calories during (and even after) the workout. If your goal is to burn fat, I highly recommend HIIT. You can torch more calories in less time. One study showed that you can burn up to 15 calories a minute with some types of HIIT. Now the people in that study were really pushing hard, but it may be something you can work up to. The great thing about it is that high-intensity is relative. Someone who is just starting out will obviously feel that a workout is hard at less intensity than someone who is very fit, but it's still hard for you, and that's what matters. Plus, good news for EveryGirls: We seem to push harder and, therefore get more out of HIIT, than men do! You don't want every workout you do to be HIIT, but try rotating it in.

STRENGTH TRAINING: This, as you know, involves exercises that require you to move some weight around, whether it be dumbbells, barbells, medicine balls, resistance bands, or even your own body

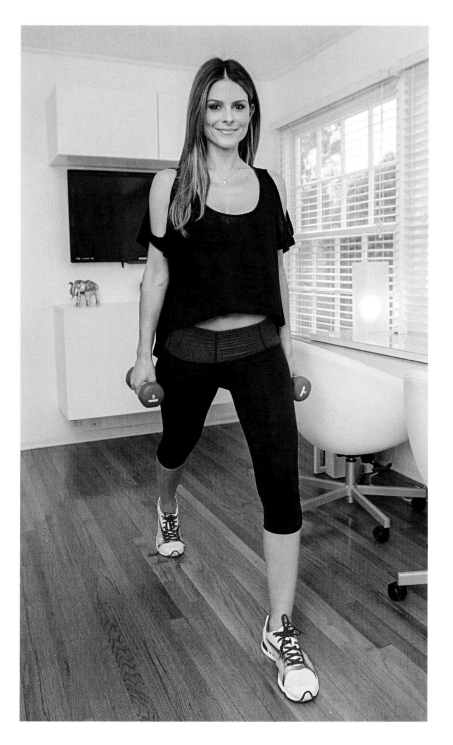

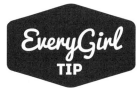

SWEAT IT OUT

When you sweat, your body releases toxins and increases metabolism, too. It's also good for your skin and a great stress reducer!

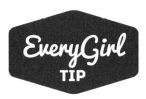

MUSCLE GROWTH

If getting seriously toned or shredded is what you're seeking, then be sure to change up your strength-training routine every few months or sooner. If you consistently do one routine, your body will acclimate, and your progress will slow or halt completely. Introduce new exercises periodically to keep challenging your body. New to working out? Start with resistance bands and then after a few months try switching to dumbbells and then barbells. After a few months of this, go back to resistance bands and so on.

weight. You push, pull, squat, lift—all to put your muscles under a little bit of stress. You may not necessarily raise your heart rate, but what you're doing is breaking down muscles and forcing them to repair themselves afterward. That's actually what builds muscle and makes muscles stronger and more resilient. Why is this important? Because muscle requires a lot of energy for your body to maintain, so it's metabolically more efficient for you to build some muscle. The more muscle you have, the more calories you burn even when you are sleeping or sitting still. It's why I think all women need to

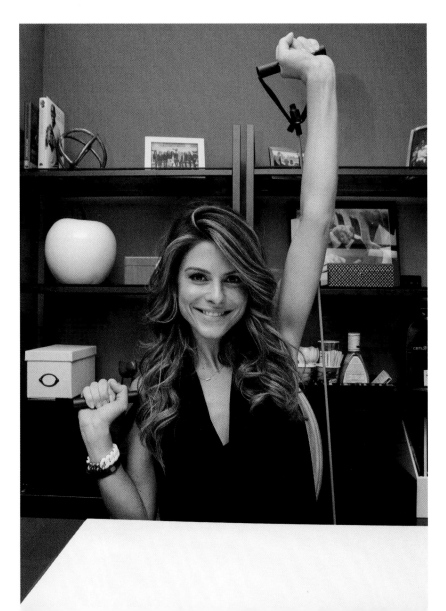

incorporate strength training into their fitness regimen. Not only will it help you get that toned, strong, and sexy look, but it will also help you burn even more calories.

RESISTANCE TRAINING: When it comes to the quickest and healthiest way to build muscle, resistance training is *the* best way to go. It's basically strength training, but strength training done right—in smooth, controlled motions. In resistance exercises, each effort is performed against a specific opposing force generated by resistance—resistance to being pushed, squeezed, stretched, or bent. For example, when you do biceps curls to build your biceps muscle, you could pull a weight or a resistance band from below your hip to the top of your shoulder and then bring it back down to your hip. For the latter part of the exercise, bringing the weight back down to your hip, you need to control the weight. Don't just drop the weight once it's at the top of your shoulder, "resist" it. By lowering the weight slowly, you are putting constant tension on the muscle, causing it to grow firmer and more defined. If you are seeking to be more toned or sculpted, you must apply that resistance.

METABOLIC WORKOUTS: This is the combo approach—where you raise your heart rate and do strength exercises at the same time. In the case of a lot of cardiovascular exercise, you may not be putting your muscles under enough strain to get sculpted. And in the case of some resistance work, you may not be raising your heart rate enough to get cardiovascular benefits. But when you combine the two, wow. You get the best of both worlds—build some muscle, work your heart. And that means you're going to burn some serious fat. This is what the popular P90X-type workouts are all about—working and challenging your body in all different ways and with all different systems. In many ways, and depending on your goals, this is often the best bang for your workout buck.

What Do I Prefer?

I do a combination of all of these. I loved my experience on *Dancing with the Stars* because dancing was indeed a cardiovascular workout, but it also worked all of my muscles so intensely—from my legs to my core. And because it blended so many different types of exercise, it's probably the reason I got in the best shape of my life. So at this stage in my journey, I like workouts that build muscle and burn calories at the same time.

When in Doubt, Choose Cardio

Reading about all these types of exercise may feel overwhelming right now. If so, start with cardio first because it is often the easiest to do, especially if it's just brisk walking, light running, swimming, bike riding, or whatever you enjoy that gets your heart pumping and oxygen into your lungs. It's also a great way to work up a sweat, ridding your body of toxins and increasing your metabolism. It's my personal number one go-to for weight loss. If I'm about to go on vacation and want to look good, I'm running on a treadmill beforehand.

Muscles Never Forget

Muscle memory is something you will want to develop—if you haven't already. By working out, as you know, you build muscle. What you may not know is that your muscles have a "mind" of their own. If you ever stop working out, your muscle tone will wane, which can be disheartening. However, thanks to muscle memory, once you resume working out, even years later, your muscles "remember" that form and tone up again rather quickly. This is why toning is worth it and why you shouldn't get discouraged if you get out of the workout habit for a while. You can pick it right up and get your muscles back in literally a few weeks.

You Don't Need a Gym

You don't necessarily need to join a gym, and you don't need one at your house, either. Doing squats, push-ups, crunches, and other exercises that use your body weight are great ways to exercise for free, and you can do them anywhere. They are just as effective as other workouts, too. Depending on the climate, more and more people are opting for outdoor workouts or what my trainer friend Andrea Orbeck calls "urban workouts." These are geared toward outdoor environments and conditions. One of my friends does her own version of this. She walks around the block in her neighborhood while throwing a small medicine ball, then jogging to pick it up. I have many gym-free workouts for you to try in this book. I love them!

If You Want to Join a Gym . . .

Though some of you may exercise rogue—outdoors, at your office, or at different locations—it can be a great help to have a set location where you do your workouts, which is why so many people like to belong to gyms.

In general, I'm not crazy about big public gyms. I have an awkward style of running, as I said, and I am self-conscious about exercising in front of strangers. Many gyms are crowded and expensive and involve a long commute. But some are great. When Rachel and I go halfsies on a trainer, we go to a gym and it always ends up being a nice change. There's also a gym at Universal City Walk that I use because of its proximity to my job.

If there's a gym close to work or home that's not too crowded and you can afford it, joining a gym can be a great option. If you like to work out with a group of people, gyms are good because they have aerobic classes, strength-training classes, spinning classes, and more. If any of that sounds appealing and you think it will motivate you to exercise more, then by all means join a gym.

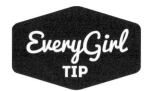

FINDING THE RIGHT GYM

If you think having a gym to go to regularly will work for you, start by taking a tour during the time of day you think you'll be using it. That way you can suss out if it's too crowded or not. Don't feel pressured by aggressive sales people; before investing in a membership, ask for a guest pass. Many gyms will let you use the facilities for a few days or even a week for free so that you can try it out. Use your trial period as an opportunity to test out the equipment and try a few classes. If you're self-conscious, you may want to try a gym that is women-only.

The Guide to Exercise Equipment

There's no doubt that you can do any kind of workout you want in your current environment. You can go for a hike or walk in the snow to burn calories and tone your legs. You can do push-ups at your desk. You can play a game of volleyball. You can take a swim in a lake or an ocean. The possibilities really are endless. But that doesn't mean there aren't all kinds of exercise equipment that can help you do the job, too, whether you use them in a gym or buy something to use at home. I can surely tell you what I like best, but as I've said, the key to establishing a good workout regimen is finding the exercises and activities that you love so that you're more likely to stick to them. Here are some of my favorites for home or at the gym.

TREADMILL: Treadmills are great for cardio and a good option when you can't run outdoors. Running on pavement can be tough on your joints. The constant pounding on your feet often leads to back, knee, and foot injury issues, but treadmills provide some "give" or "bounce," reducing the pounding. I love that I can run and watch episodes of my favorite shows while I use it, and they don't have to take up too much space. Some of the machines even fold up.

ELLIPTICAL TRAINER: The elliptical is amazing for cardio workouts, and there is virtually no pressure on your joints. It's one of the best cardio machines around.

SPINNING BIKE: A stationary bike can get your heart pumping and give you a fantastic leg workout without pounding on your joints. As is the case with other pieces of cardio equipment, you can vary the intensity so that you get an interval workout as well as

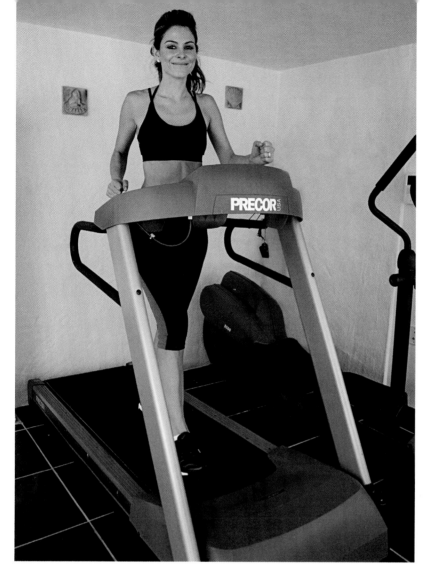

a longer, steadier workout while you watch your favorite shows.

ROWING MACHINE: Rowing machines are terrific because they provide a total-body workout. To row, you'll use your legs, your upper body, and your core and get great cardio, too.

BOWFLEX: It provides great resistance training, has a wide range of exercises, and is safe to use when working out alone. Both women and men like it and it's a great, safe, space-saving unit.

POWERTEC: Guys who really want to push heavy free weights safely alone will love it. However, it's simple and safe for us gals to use, too. It offers a wide variety of exercises that work every muscle. Plus it doesn't take up much space, considering everything that it does.

DUAL-STACK MACHINES: These machines are space-saving and offer smooth-form exercises for muscles with good resistance. You can exercise every part of your body in a safe way, and they're becoming more popular in gyms across the country. It's what

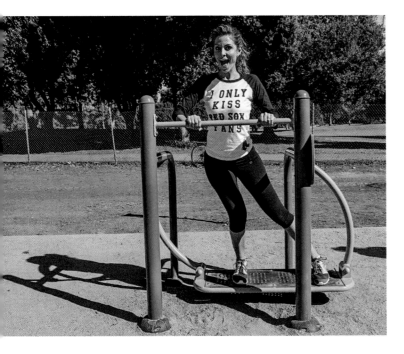

Harley Pasternak recommended I get for our home gym. Incidentally, Harley designed the used one I bought on Craigslist. They're also available at sporting goods stores or large department stores. Some are sturdier and better made than others, of course. Visit the stores and test them out for yourself.

DOOR GYMS: These are similar to resistance bands, but they are units that hang on the back of a door, where it stays out of sight. The exercises you can do on the Weider X-Factor Door Gym are similar to the ones you do on the Bowflex and the stack machines. It's easy to install, doesn't require drilling, and sells for under a hundred dollars. I have one at my parents' house and one in my production office.

OUTDOOR EQUIPMENT: Recently, in Los Angeles, many parks and playgrounds have been outfitted with outdoor exercise equipment. PlayCore is a company that installs the particular type used in our neighborhoods, which works a number of different body parts and also helps add variety to your

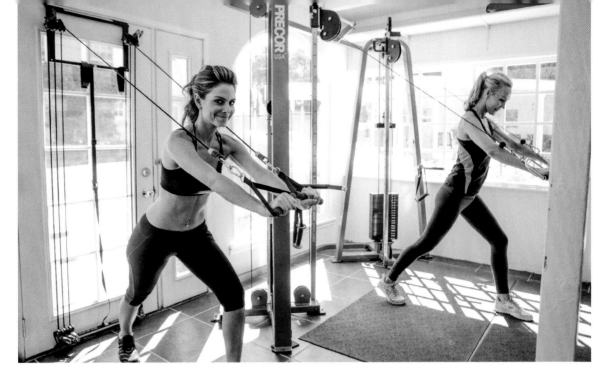

cardio workout. PlayCore also helps build stronger communities around the world by advancing recreation through research and educational programs, and building public gyms in parks and recreation areas for towns across the country. It's encouraging to see people of all ages and fitness levels using the equipment! To learn more about bringing outdoor fitness parks to your community, log on to *playcore.com/fitness*.

IPODS: Whether it's an iPod or an iPhone or any smartphone in general, there are few greater tools in your workout arsenal. Music, audio books, and podcasts all keep you engaged while you are working out. Sometimes I'll have my iPod attached to speakers, and other times I'll use my headphones. Sometimes I'll listen to music from a special workout playlist I created. Other times, I listen to podcasts. I can't tell you how many fans of AfterBuzz TV write to tell us how much they love listening to AfterBuzz podcasts while working out! They'll watch their favorite TV show, then download and listen to an AfterBuzz recap/aftershow, which makes the workout go by that much faster. Either way, it's another effective piece of equipment.

↑ I love that we are getting the same workout on two very different priced machines. The over-the-door gym is around $100 and the other goes for $2,000. .

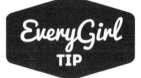

IPOD ESSENTIALS

I know that for many music is an essential part of a good workout. If you keep your workout playlist on your smartphone, consider getting an armband for your phone, it will keep your phone safe and your hands free to move freely. Another option is a an iPod Shuffle, they're tiny, the same size as stamp, hold plenty of songs, and clip right to your waist.

The Bs of Fitness: Bells, Balls, and Bands

The essence of this book is about gaining health and fitness when you don't have the time or money. I know some of the above items are no more pricey than a gym membership, but they could still be too costly for you. The Bs of fitness are tools that are cheap, space-saving, and extremely effective. If it makes you feel any better, I happen to use all of the equipment below!

MEDICINE BALLS: Medicine balls are especially wonderful if you like working out in a group or with a partner, because you can use them to provide extra resistance in some abs exercises. (Here's an example: Lie on your back with your feet on the floor, arms extended overhead, and hold a medicine ball in your hands. Crunch your torso up, and at the top of the movement toss the ball to your buddy. Wait for her to throw it back, then curl back down, and

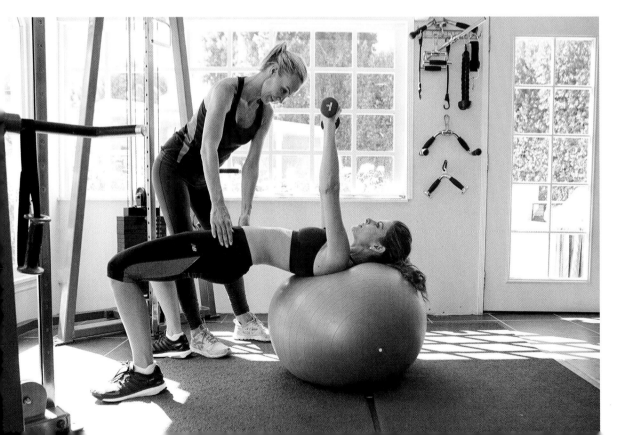

repeat.) You can also use them for multi-muscle exercises, such as squatting and then tossing the ball up toward the ceiling as you rise. These are great total-body combo exercises that give you an efficient workout in a short amount of time. I love doing ab work with balls. For me, it feels less like a workout and more like playing a game.

STABILITY BALLS: Stability balls are large, inflatable rubber balls that are used for strength training, stretching, and core muscle exercises. They are excellent tools that have a wide range of uses and benefits. Most stability balls come with workout routine manuals to show you what exercises you can do. You'd be surprised what great results you get from using them. I have a friend who had back problems, and her doctor advised her to use a stability ball in place of her desk chair. Taking the advice, she sits on one while at her desk. It keeps her back straight and helps build her core.

RESISTANCE BANDS: They're wonderful for travel because they're small, light, and can fit into

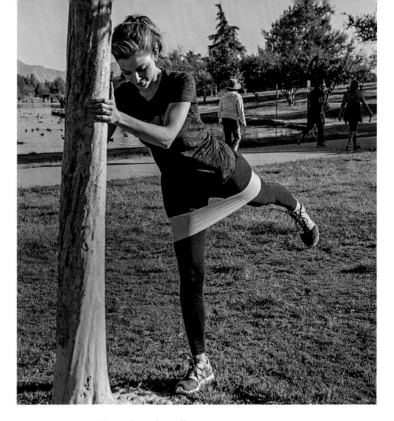

any carry-on, these bands will allow you to do strength workouts if you're on the go. By providing resistance, the bands serve a similar purpose as dumbbells as you pull and push them in different directions to work different muscles. Kev and I use them all the time.

BLOCKS: When I say blocks, I mean stepping blocks—ones you can step up and down on for exercise. They are great space-saving pieces. There are also yoga blocks, which you can use to make it easier to get into different poses.

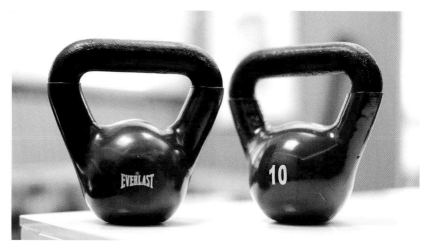

DUMBBELLS, KETTLEBELLS: Of course, these are standard pieces of equipment in most gyms, and they're a great way to work your muscles because of the infinite number of moves you can do with them. Because most of us are not power-lifting, one to three pairs of light bells will do the trick.

BARBELLS: I have a couple of weighted bars that I keep in my bedroom, and office. You can do almost every exercise with them. Harley Pasternak, incidentally, has a product called the Harley Bar that collapses and fits into a tiny bag. It's another great weapon in the no-time, no-money, no-space battle for fitness.

BOXING EQUIPMENT: Punching a heavy bag is one of the best ways to get your heart rate up and develop strength. If you're looking for a piece of equipment that's efficient and good for both men and women, this may be it. We had one for several years, and it was great. Add in a jump rope and some dumbbells and you can create a mini-circuit that will get your heart pumping fast—two minutes of punching, two minutes of jumping rope, and then a couple of strength exercises. Repeat that circuit for twenty minutes, and you'll have worked out like a champ. And it's a great way to get some aggression out!

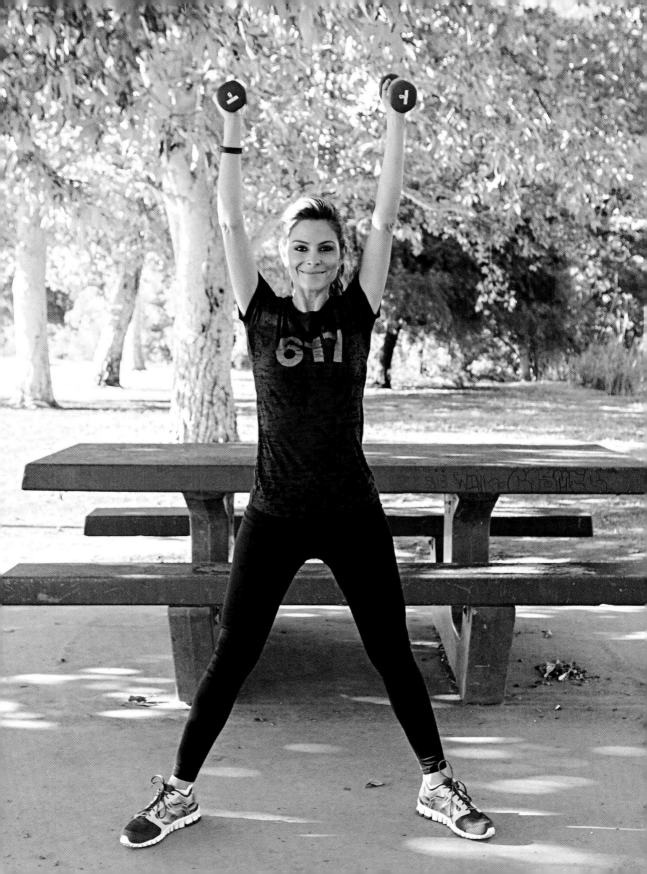

Creating Your Home Gym

If you want to set up your own gym, whether it's in the basement, garage, or just in the corner of a room there are many possibilities. What equipment you buy and where you set things up depends on what you can afford and what space you have. The amazing news is that with the equipment available today you can get a great workout in the smallest of spaces.

If you don't think you need all the things that a regular gym has to offer, I would seriously consider working out at home. For the Every-Girl who's trying to cram everything into her life, I thoroughly recommend it. The convenience can't be beat. You can roll out of bed and work out, or work out when you get home as dinner is cooking or while you catch up on your favorite TV series. Commuting to the gym and getting dressed takes time, sometimes up to an hour when you add it all up. It doesn't seem like much, but over time it is. Plus, what if it rains or snows? Working out at home minimizes these and other obstacles. The more obstacles, the less inclined you'll be to work out. Also, you'll save on gym memberships by investing in your own equipment.

Kev and I have a gym at home, but truthfully, Kev's the one who mostly uses it. Honestly, my home gym is pretty big, and I don't need a gym the size of the one Kev and I have in our home, nor do you. I do most of my workouts with stuff like mats, balls, and bands in places like my bedroom, office, or backyard. In the last house we lived in, though, I did use a home gym. The house was small, but there was a small shed in the backyard. I painted the walls, threw down a rug and a boom box, hung up a mirror and a small TV and was off and working out. Some things to consider if you want to create your home gym:

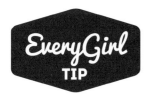

EveryGirl TIP

BUY USED GYM EQUIPMENT!

Many people buy equipment and then never use it. Some get bored of it. Others, including gym owners, just want to upgrade their equipment. Places like Craigslist and eBay are great resources to find amazing deals on workout equipment. Local gyms may even be willing to sell you older pieces of equipment at a steep discount. Kev and I scored our used dual stack machine for $800. New ones sell for over $2000!

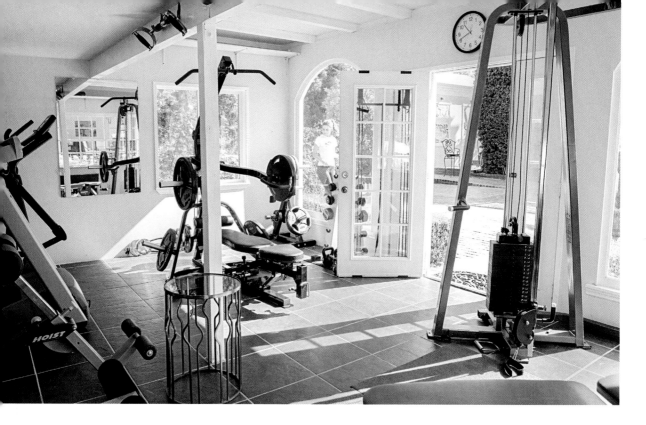

LOCATION: Depending on climates, basements, spare rooms, and garages all make great gyms. My mom uses her basement, and I have multiple friends who go the spare room or garage route. It's a great luxury to have a separate area, but again, it's not necessary. You can put an elliptical in the corner of your bedroom or TV room, for instance.

ON THE WALLS: If you have the space and money, I'd like to see you hang a large mirror or two. Hell, if you have the money you can make an entire wall a mirror.

It's not a vanity thing. It's a great way to watch yourself as you exercise in order to keep good form. Mirrors are relatively easy to hang, and places like Target, Home Depot, Lowe's, and Walmart have great ones that are affordable. Or, you could hit up a mirror and glass company in your area. You may be surprised how inexpensive a large sheet of mirror is to buy and install.

I love hanging inspirational quotes on the walls. You can also put up some great pictures of yourself at your target weight or photos of other people that will inspire you. Stuff like this can keep you motivated to keep going when you want to quit.

FLOORING: Area commercial rugs are available at stores like Target, Walmart, Home Depot, and Lowe's. Also available at Home Depot and Loew's are rubber floor squares that interconnect to create one big exercise mat. They are super-easy to clean, give you that professional gym feel, and provide great support for your feet. The padding is also great for working with dumbbells or weights because if dropped, they may damage your floors.

ENTERTAINMENT: TVs, DVRs, and even game systems can be great additions to a home gym. I have an old small flat-panel TV that has a built-in DVD player. I also have used a DVR through my cable service, programmed to record my favorite series. With these items, cardio workouts, particularly on treadmills, bikes, and elliptical machines, go by faster and you get to catch up on your movies and TV shows. My TV was

seventy-nine dollars and the mount was under twenty dollars. It's a luxury, yes, but if that's what it takes to motivate you to workout, it's not a huge investment. If you don't have cable or satellite, you can use a laptop or an iPad. Also, game boxes like Wii and Xbox can also be used to play music, videos, or even games that involve physical activity.

EQUIPMENT: If you have the space for a variety of tools, gadgets, and machines and the money to pay for them, and that's what it takes for you to be motivated, then have at it. If you have at least a space of about eight square feet, then I suggest you designate one area for cardio (like a stationary bike, elliptical, or treadmill) and one for strength training (like dumbbells, a bench, mat, or ball). As I mentioned before, you can create an excellent workout space by buying used equipment on eBay or Craigslist like Kev and I did. There is always an abundance available.

The Bedroom Gym

I didn't always have a separate space for a gym. In my apartment, my home gym was a corner of my bedroom. It was all the space I had, but it was extremely convenient, cost-effective, and yielded great results. I stored my sneakers, dumbbells, resistance bands, and yoga mat in an under-bed storage container (the type that's used to store long rolls of wrapping paper). When I wanted to work out, I'd slide the container out and take what I needed, and when I was done, I'd put the equipment back and slide it neatly under the bed. I set up a treadmill within viewing distance of an old TV; although today, I'd probably watch TV on an iPad or a laptop. And I'd tuck my feet under my dresser to do situps. Just think: You can wake up just twenty minutes earlier, roll out of bed and to get in the workout you need.

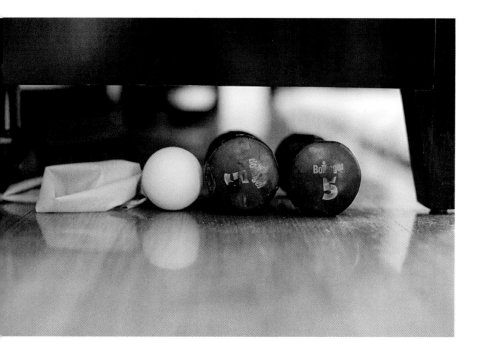

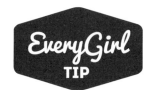

HOME GYM FENG SHUI
The key is to set up your workout space in a place you'll really enjoy using and spending time in. I recently visited some friends who set aside a room as their "gym." Frankly, it was depressing. The room was dark, there was nothing on the walls, the TV was in a totally different direction than the treadmill. I didn't say anything because they seemed excited, but I knew there was no way they were going to want to work out there. I asked them how many times they had used it, and they were like, "Well, I have my bag in there; I'm going to start tomorrow."
Sadly, the last time I checked, tomorrow never came. If you're going to do it, set it up don't go halfway. Do it right so that you will be motivated to use it.

Workout Videos

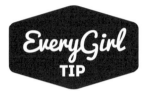

CHECK OUT ANDREA'S WEBSITE

Andrea has some great workout videos on her website *andreaorbeck.com*. From how to get super-model thighs (she should know, she's Heidi Klum's trainer) to prenatal fitness, she covers it all.

As I'm kicking all the tires and laying out all the options for you, I have to praise the workout video. It's the very best tool I can suggest. For around ten bucks, you are essentially getting a trainer to guide you through a workout that provides both motivation and instruction. The workout can be done in your home, generally with inexpensive equipment. As Jack LaLanne recommended changing up your workouts every thirty days, with videos you can do that easily. If you have a few, you can rotate them and you won't get bored as quickly. If all you did was cut back on portions and follow workout videos a few times a week, I'd say great job!

Whether you play them on the TV in your bedroom or living room or on your computer, workout videos are amazing and, I feel, underrated in terms of achieving fitness. But there are many on the market, so I want to list some of my favorites.

HARLEY PASTERNAK, *HARLEY'S 5-FACTOR WORKOUT*: Harley, whom I have mentioned many times, is not only my friend but also one of the most knowledgeable authorities on the science of diet and fitness. His video delivers a fast and effective workout for you as well as your boyfriend or partner. I love it!

JILLIAN MICHAELS: Jillian is also my friend and has so many great videos. You can't go wrong with any of them, but I especially like **30 Day Shred.** It's a full-body 20-minute workout you can do for a month or longer because it has workouts at different intensity levels, so it works with you as you get fitter. For a little more intensity, you may want to try her **Grab Weights and Slim Down** series. All you need are resistance bands; a pair each of 3-, 5-, and 10-pound dumbbells; and a yoga mat. It's a three-month program designed to burn fat and build muscle in just thirty minutes a workout. If you're into yoga or Pilates, Jillian has a great video for you as well.

PUSSYCAT DOLLS WORKOUT:
I know from experience what dancing can do for your body. Another great friend, Pussycat Dolls creator and world-famous choreographer, Robin Antin developed this fun and sexy dance workout. Along with the girls from the Pussycat Lounge Review, Robin will show you simple but striking signature dance moves you can do along to hit Pussycat Dolls songs. It's a great way to dance your way to a lean and toned body.

P90X: P90X has become one of the most popular forms of exercise. The series of videos enables you to get a great workout with very little equipment. You're always changing routines, changing the way you exercise, and using all kinds of cool movements—from classic strength

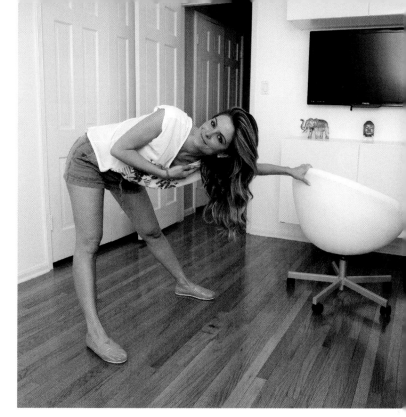

moves to yoga-inspired moves to moves that even elite athletes do. P90X is based on the idea that in order for you to get stronger (and lose weight), your muscles need to be confused.

ANDREA ORBECK,
PREGNANCY SCULPT:
For those of you expecting, I wouldn't put you in anyone else's hands. Using her famous "minute moves," Andrea helps expectant moms stay fit during pregnancy and bounce back into their skinny jeans afterward. Also check out **Supermodel Butt and Thighs.**

Pick Your Exercise Treats

I like to sprinkle in exercise treats—that is, exercises that I may not get to do very often but that I love doing. You may love Zumba or swimming but just can't work it in that often—maybe because of the time the class is offered or because getting to the pool isn't very convenient. That's okay—but don't give up on them for good just because you can't make them your go-to workouts. Consider them activities you do as a treat every once in a while. The variety will help your body get better results, because changing routines has been proven to do so. It also stimulates you and keeps you from getting bored. I encourage you to experiment and make up your own list of favorite once-in-a-while treat activities. Here are mine:

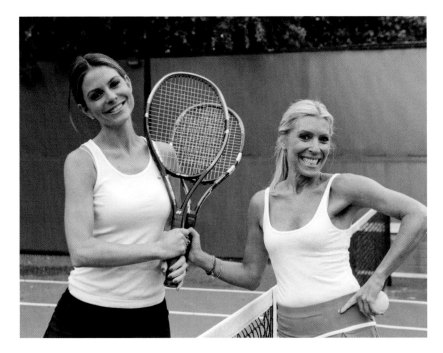

THE EVERYGIRL'S GUIDE TO DIET AND FITNESS

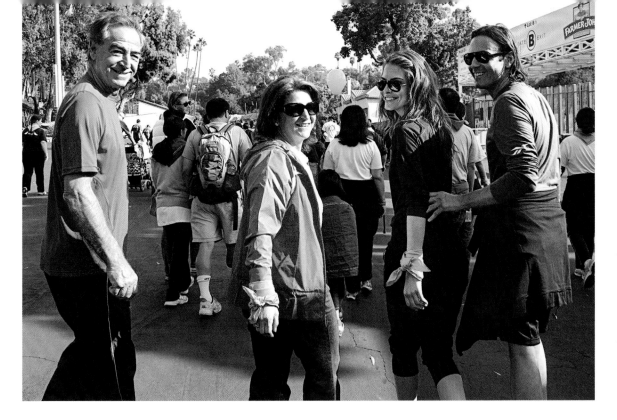

↑ I love road races! We try to do as many as we can like this L.A. Cancer Challenge. Great double-whammy!

ROAD RACES: I love participating in road races, like 5Ks and 10Ks. They're manageable distances, since I don't have a lot of free time to train for something like a marathon, and they give you a sense of accomplishment. It forces you to go outside and join like-minded people on a mission. Many have a charitable component, so it makes you feel like you're doing something not for you alone but for the greater good. I sometimes freak at the starting time since it's often really early, but once I get there, I feel empowered and excited to be exercising in the fresh air. Also, I love the challenge. I find people I want to beat throughout the race. I keep pushing myself to run faster and get ahead of them. I'm always inspired to see older people running, too, and then I think, I want to be like them at their age. So sign up for as many as you can . . . and bring friends. Short races are a great way to socialize, do something charitable, get a great workout in, and maybe even meet someone cute! And remember: It's okay if you can't keep up with the pace of others. Feel free to walk and jog portions.

SPIN CLASSES: I never thought I would like spinning because I hate riding the bike at the gym. But then I decided to host a spin class for charity and realized how amazing it was. I always say that good music inspires me to work out longer and harder than I expected, and good spin classes have incredible music. The music intensifies to get you through the tough parts, the instructors keep you pumped, and they keep the lights off so it feels like a nightclub. What I love about this is, nobody is looking at you, so you can go at your own pace and not be embarrassed. The time flew by, and it was a pretty inspiring experience. You feel like you are pushing yourself to levels you never knew you could attain. And there was something really cathartic about it. The kind of feeling you have when you go to church. Or at least it felt like that for me.

YOGA MORNINGS: Often, I try to get ready a few minutes earlier in the morning so that I have time for a quick yoga workout. The key is, I don't make it a big deal. I don't need workout gear, and I do it for whatever time I have available. I have posted pictures of me in a sundress doing yoga on Twitter. I do a few poses, breathe in the fresh air, and end it with saying something positive out loud like "Today is going to be a great day." These yoga mornings make me feel like at least I'm doing something positive. Breathing is important. And positivity is definitely a must as well. When it gets cold, I do yoga indoors. It's not as fun as being outside with the sun, but it still serves its purpose.

"Health, fitness and dieting is really all about one thing: Confidence—and gaining more and more of it every day.."

Tara Kraft, former editor in chief, SHAPE Magazine

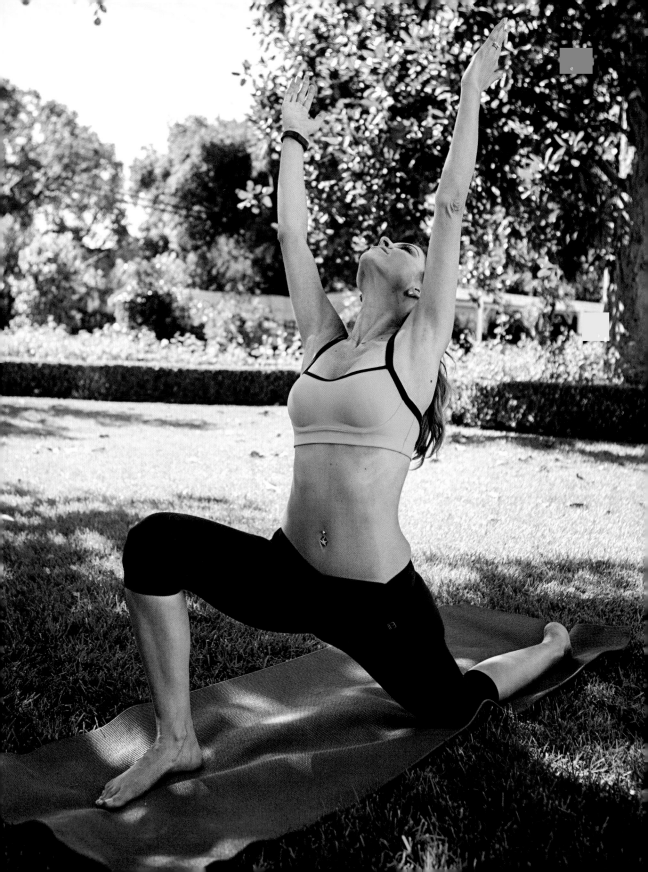

How do you stay motivated to eat right and exercise?

I think the motivation for me is feeling, not looking, a certain way. A lot of people say, "I want to lose weight and get healthy and I want to slim down." For me, it's not because I want to look healthy per se. It's because I want to feel my best. When I eat healthily, I feel better. That doesn't mean I'm not going to have a cheat and indulge myself in truffle fries once in a blue moon.

What is the healthiest diet change you've made?

My biggest accomplishment with food is what I completely eliminated: I don't use salt when I cook; I don't put it on foods. At a restaurant, I ask for low-sodium or salt-free dishes. Believe it or not, once I got rid of salt, I started tasting the food, and it tasted way better.

How do you stay in shape?

I believe workouts have to be versatile—you don't want your muscles to get used to the workout you're doing. That's when you stop seeing results. I like to constantly mix workouts up. I like to do Bikram yoga in the heat—I like the heat; it opens up muscles and joints. I like SoulCycle—forty-five minutes of intense cycling while working your arms with weights. It's workout torture, but then you feel incredible afterward. I love classes. I realize I'm way better working out in class because I get distracted alone and my ADD kicks in. I always mix it up.

When you need to prep for a photo shoot, a special event, or the red carpet, what do you do?

If I have a bikini shoot where I need to be in certain shape, I work out intensely every single day for about two weeks. Then a week before the shoot, I start slowing down. Muscles actually swell up

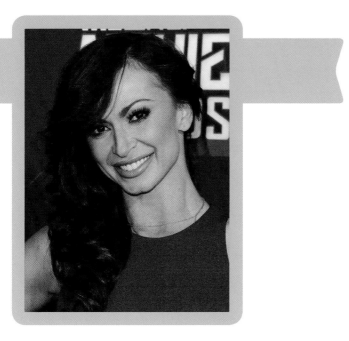

when you work out like crazy. I still do yoga and stretching. I eat watermelon—it's a diuretic, so it helps your body get rid of excess water. A day before the shoot, I have a boiled chicken breast and boiled sweet potato—it takes more water out of you, and you will look ripped that day. And your muscles go schoooooooom.

What does your diet look like on a typical day?

Normally I start the day with scrambled egg whites with spinach, and if I have asparagus from the night before, I'll throw that in. If not, I start with a smoothie with kale, pineapple, and berries, and I take that with me and sip throughout the day because it's filling, healthy, easy, and it's delicious, too. I'm not a big fan of having a lot of snacks during the day, because I need to move a lot and need to dance a lot. So I might do something like trail mix or hummus with celery or baby carrots. When I get home, my easy go-to is grilled chicken breast—you can make it in five or seven minutes—and a spinach salad with cranberries and walnuts. It's healthy and delicious. And I always have a glass of red wine.

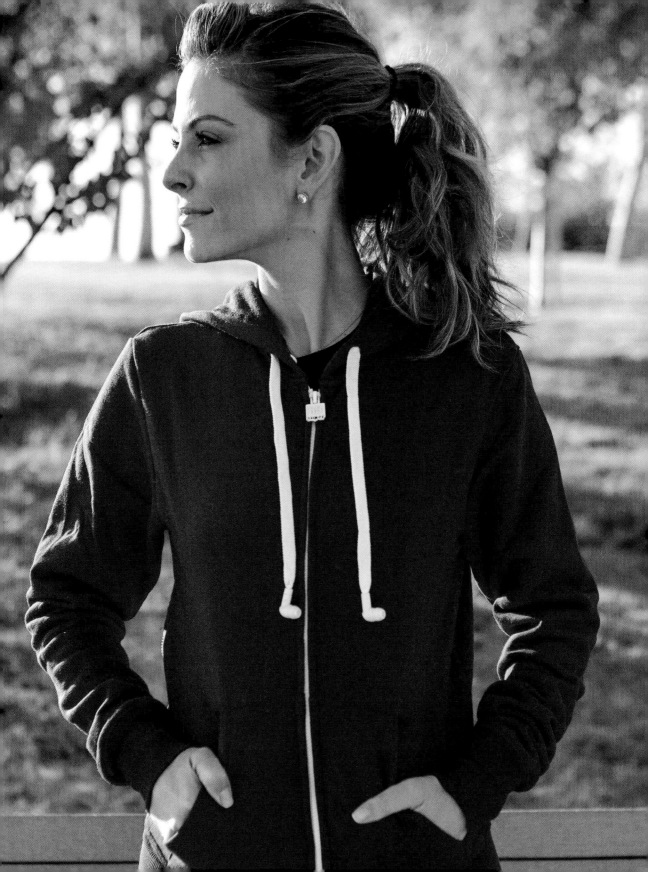

Chapter 11

EveryGirl's Excuse-Proof Life

I've made no secret that this book centers around overcoming the two big roadblocks people face when trying to lose weight or get healthy—time and money. I hope that I've done enough to help you overcome those obstacles. However, I know that there are other issues that might interfere with your attempts to get healthier and fitter out there. Let me give you some solutions to the most common ones.

PROBLEM:
Changing My Whole Life Around Feels So Daunting.

SOLUTION: Every time we have changes to make in the office, rather than spook everyone and tell them that big changes are coming, we'll say, "It's nothing big . . . just a few minor adjustments." You might want to adopt the same mentality. The tricks and tips I've given you so far are really just a few minor adjustments, if you think about it. But guess what? Over time, all these tiny adjustments add up to big changes. If you think of it that way and remember that you don't have to do a 180—it feels much more doable.

PROBLEM:
But I Just Love Cheesesteaks!

SOLUTION: Hey, I love them, too! If you look at how I ate when I lost the weight, you'll see that I didn't deprive myself. I still ate pizza and sweets. I just cut back on it all. Don't think that you have to give up everything you love. You're just cutting back. Strive to follow the 75/25 plan. Over time, you'll have a cleaner diet overall.

PROBLEM:
I Can't Cook, So Takeout Is the Easiest Option.

SOLUTION: Well, I hope that my recipes will help with that problem. And yes, sometimes, busy schedules dictate that you'll have to eat out, but even unhealthy places do have healthy options. When in doubt, order grilled chicken and a salad with light dressing on the side, and use only as much dressing as you need. I highly recommend you invest in a cooking class. Check out your local community colleges. They often offer some continuing education classes or check out some YouTube videos. You can even barter with a kitchen-savvy friend to teach you. The more control you have over your food, the greater chance you'll have of making this whole thing work for you.

Also, if you make a few of my recipes on a Sunday evening and combine them into meals, you'll save time. You can eat something healthy every night of the week, but you don't have to cook every night. That's what I do. If you opened my fridge on any given day, you'd see that it was full of recipes from this book or my last book. It makes eating well so easy and tasty to boot!

PROBLEM:

I Just Need Something Sweet to Get Me Out of That Afternoon Slump.

SOLUTION: What does the rest of your diet look like *before* you hit that slump? I bet it's full of sugars and refined carbs. If you cut back on them or replaced them earlier in the day, you probably wouldn't feel tired or crabby around 3 or 4 p.m. As I said previously, refined carbs spike your blood sugar, but then lead to a big crash, which is why you feel blah, and then you reach for more refined carbs or sugar to pick you up again. Break the cycle by trying to have healthier carbs and more fiber and protein earlier in the day. If you still feel like you need a pick-me-up in the afternoon, it's better to have water or some of the healthy snacks mentioned earlier. Even better: Take a short power walk, or do a few minutes of stretching at your desk.

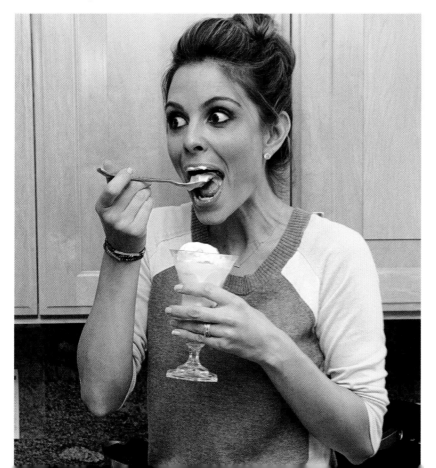

PROBLEM:
I Don't Have Time to Do a Lot of Food Prep.

SOLUTION: One of my favorite kitchen tools is a Magic Bullet that makes shakes and smoothies. In the simplest form, just add protein powder, skim milk, and a few fruits, and you've just created a wonderful meal in seconds. But the beauty of these blenders are that you can create all kinds of healthy and delicious concoctions with fruit and vegetables. One warning, though: Some people get so excited about all the things they can add to a drink that they add so many ingredients and turn what should be a healthy smoothie into a calorie-bomb. To add volume to healthy smoothies, just add more ice or water—it allows you to fill up a little more without having to load up on calories. A lot of people love to add kale and spinach, too, to get more nutrients, because they blend in easily without altering the taste of the other ingredients.

In addition, you don't need to make complicated stuff. My bean patties take ten minutes to prepare as do so many other items included in this book.

PROBLEM:
But I Hate Vegetables!

SOLUTION: There are lots of ways to add flavor to them without junking them up (cheese sauce does not count). For example, you can try drizzling them with a little olive oil and sprinkling them with your favorite spice (garlic or crushed red pepper, perhaps?), and then roasting them. Roasting makes veggies sweeter. Lots of people also like eating raw veggies with a little hummus. If you really can't stomach them, then try sneaking a little into a healthy smoothie—add a little kale or spinach and you'll get the nutrients without the taste. I encourage you to give my mom's vegetable recipes a try though. I have friends who hate cooking, but love our easy-to-make recipes so much that they find themselves making these veggie dishes almost daily!

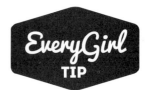

KEEP A YOGA MAT AND THERA-BAND BY YOUR BED
I try to commit to a few stretches at night and a few leg exercises by morning from the various options I provided later in the book. Remember, its all about baby steps.

PROBLEM:

I Am So Exhausted from Working All Day and Taking Care of My Family That I Can't Even Think About Doing a 15-Minute Workout.

SOLUTION: As I said, I just find other ways to incorporate working out into my day. Taking the stairs at every turn is the obvious option. On set, I'll randomly do calf raises. In the shower, I'll do the same (be careful not to slip). While cooking, when I'm waiting for something to boil or simmer, I'll do some squats or push-ups on the counter. I just find ways to include working out into my daily duties and to do something as opposed to doing nothing. And remember, if you curb and control *what* and *how much* you eat, heavy-duty workouts won't be as crucial.

PROBLEM:

Everybody in My Family Is This Size and Shape, So This Is How I'm Supposed to Be.

SOLUTION: I think this is something that many women believe. They look at how their mothers looked at their age and—good or bad—that's how they think they're going to look, too. While genetics is a strong influencer of weight issues, more and more research is showing that the genetics can be out-muscled by the way you eat and the way you live. Now, does that mean you can change your inherent shape or the tendency to gain weight in a certain place? No, but it does mean that most of us can control our size through making dietary changes and exercising. I think just knowing that—and not using genetics as the reason why you can't lose weight—can be empowering enough to take a chance. You can use genetics as an explanation, but not as an excuse.

PROBLEM:
I'm Injured.

SOLUTION: First and foremost, if you have an injury that hurts you enough to sideline you from exercise, you absolutely need to figure out the source of the problem—and then the best course of action. If your body needs rest, you need to take the rest. Just rushing back from an injury will only lead to more (and more serious) injuries, so you'll be setting yourself up for longer-term problems. But you also don't need to think that injury has to mean inactivity. Depending on your situation, you may be able to do some type of exercise to maintain a low level of fitness while the hurt body part heals. If you have a foot injury and can't run, try swimming or biking or doing an upper-body workout. This can be a challenging time, and it can be easy to fall into the trap of letting yourself go while you wait for your trouble spot to recover, but I encourage you to talk to your doctor and physical therapist about what options you have. Take the time to heal, but keep your "mind in the state of possibility" that there's usually *something* you can do. After *Dancing with the Stars,* I was determined to keep my newly toned body in shape. However, I was *so* broken. I hired a trainer for a day who helped me develop a workout plan that involved mat Pilates-based moves that protected my feet.

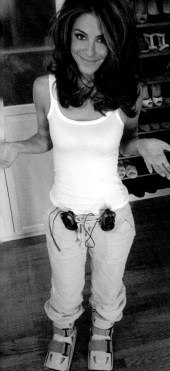

↓ Here I am during *Dancing with the Stars* with my bone stimulators and my protective boots. I did everything I could to stay in the game.

THE EVERYGIRL'S GUIDE TO DIET AND FITNESS

PROBLEM:

Everybody Around Me Has Unhealthy Habits, and I Can't Find Anyone Who Wants to Do What I'm Doing.

SOLUTION: Don't use this as a reason why you can't engage in healthy eating and regular exercise. Nobody around you? Turn to groups online. Find blogs you like of people who think the way you do, or join online communities with message boards or Facebook groups. Also, recall some of the activities I recommended: Races, Zumba, volleyball, dancing, roller-skating; doing these group-based activities can help you meet like-minded folks. And just so you know, I didn't have anyone at first, either. At the time, many of my friends were engaging in unhealthy activities, and my new plan didn't jibe with that. It was hard to deal with, but I followed the advice I've given you in this book. The general rule is to do your best to avoid situations that will make it difficult for you to stick with your game plan. It's not easy, but I'm living proof that it can be done.

PROBLEM:

Sweat Is Just Gross.

SOLUTION: Sweat helps rid your body of toxins and has other benefits. But workouts and sweating are not always convenient for us women. We can't just hop in the shower, put on our clothes, and be back at work after a lunchtime run. I go back to my "anything is better than nothing" rule. A walk is better than sitting at the desk. So are a few push-ups or a little stretch or some other small activity that can keep your body moving without producing a gallon of sweat. So do something. And like I said earlier: I always carry baby wipes with me. They're not high-powered enough to handle a heavy-duty session, but they're just enough to handle a little mini power walk up the office stairs.

PROBLEM:
I'm on the Road a Lot.

SOLUTION: This all comes down to preparation. Yes, there will be times when you may have to rely on fast food, airport food, or hole-in-the-wall food. Most of them do have healthy choices. When in doubt, think grilled chicken and lots of vegetables. But if you are prepared, you can do even better. Are you in a situation where you can pack snacks? Fruits, nuts, string cheese, whole-wheat crackers, or healthy energy bars can keep you full through-out the day. Can you stay in hotels with small fridges in the room? If so, take a quick trip to a local supermarket to get some essen-tials so that you don't have to hit the hotel buffet every morning. You can also pack a resistance band to work out in your room if the motel or hotel doesn't have a gym. The point is that, yes, your environment changes, but you can adjust to that. And taking just a little bit of time on the front end in terms of preparation will help a lot. Tip: Have the hotel remove any minibar temptations prior to your arrival to avoid temptation. When I travel, I hit what-ever local market there is and pick up water, bananas, almonds, and Greek yogurt for my room. Where there's a will there's a way.

PROBLEM:
I Had a Really (Really, Really) Bad Day.

SOLUTION: Remember you have that 25 percent food cush-ion—go ahead and indulge in some comfort food if it will help. While it may not be the healthiest option, sometimes that comfort can help us through a tough day or a tough hour. But when those hours and days turn to weeks and months, and we rely on sugary snack foods to manage the stress, that's when the comfort turns to conflict. That's when the accumulated effect of stress—and our response to it—add up to an unhealthy body. For me, when I've had a bad day, maybe I'll have a beer or some kind of fried appetizer. But I have just one, really taking time to enjoy it, and then I stop. And I know that deep down, it's a bad cycle to get into—and if I really want to be healthy, I need to figure my way out of whatever problem I'm having. I then realize there are fewer natural depression busters as good as exercise and that a good workout is a great way to turn a bad day around.

PROBLEM:
But, But, But . . . It's Vacation. It's a Holiday. Heck, It's the Weekend!

SOLUTION: I'm the last person to tell you that you need to eat perfectly while celebrating good times. My strategy is to enjoy the things I really love while either being aware of not going all-out crazy or being sure I can make up for it in some other way. I do try to stick to my 75/25 guideline even while traveling, but there are ways to deal with it, should my intentions go astray. A good countermove to vacation indulgence is to make an effort to spend some time walking on the beach and not just lounging on it. Walk a lot, go sightseeing on foot, try to work in a little routine at the hotel gym. For parties and such, get in an extra-hard workout on a morning you know you're going to have the family over for a cookout. Does it negate every calorie? No, but it does help. And I'm not saying that you should have workouts hanging over your head during every holiday and vacation, but I *am* saying that if it is an option, why not try to do a little some-

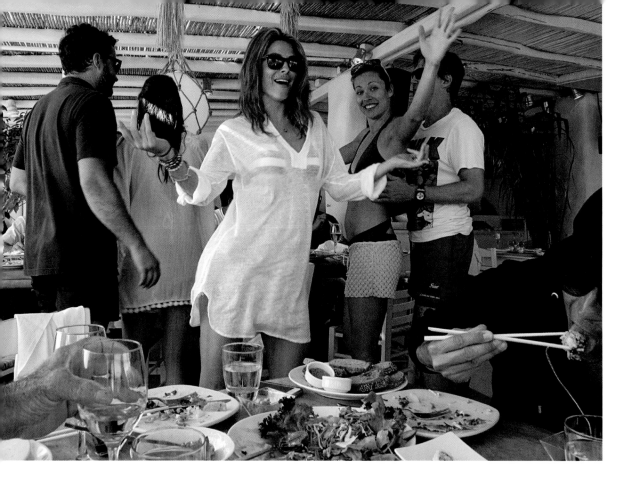

↑ Dancing with my
goddaughter's parents
Marietta and Leon on vacation
in Mykonos with my family.
A little tip: If you're bikini top
doesn't have any padding,
you can make a small cut
into the inside lining and insert
cups you've purchase. A dry-
cleaner's tailor can do this for you
as well for as little as $10.

thing? You can also try cutting back your food by 10 percent for a few weeks prior to the trip.

Tip: Want to curb jet lag when traveling? Hit the gym for a work-out as soon as you land. It works!

PROBLEM:
Exercise Is So Boring.

SOLUTION: With workouts, it's important to eliminate any obstacle in my path but also to incorporate every boost, every bit of help I can find to motivate me. Whatever way I need to trick my brain or pump myself up into eating right or exercising, I do it. Below are some of those things that I implement.

CREATE A PLAYLIST: I listen to music when I exercise, and there's nothing like a good beat to up my intensity. Take the time to download songs that will pump you up and get you through your workout. Be sure to create a few playlists so that you can switch them up; that way they never get stale. On that note, I intentionally only allow myself to listen to these playlists when working out. I keep them off-limits so I don't burn out on those songs and so I look forward to hearing them. Knowing I have a great playlist to listen to actually makes me excited to work out just to hear the music. My favorite workout songs are "Welcome to the Jungle" by Guns n' Roses or anything by Bon Jovi. And there's also nothing like a little Gloria Estefan to get me going.

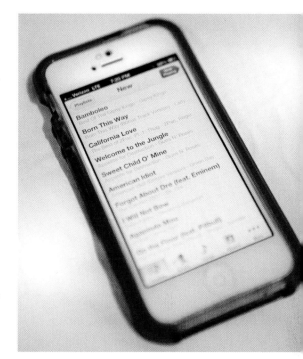

PUT AN INSPIRATION PHOTO ON YOUR FRIDGE: This could be a picture of you at a time you looked your best. I do it. It's a great motivator. Or post a picture of someone whose body you admire. You don't want her body per se, you want *your* best body. But there's nothing wrong with a little inspiration. Visualizing your goals really helps. And so does posting your inspiration photo on the fridge. Every time you go to open the door, it will make you think and may be just the thing to dissuade you from overindulging.

CREATE AN INSPIRATION WALL: I have a wall in my office of amazing quotes from great people, such as "You never lose unless you quit!" and other inspirational sayings. There are companies that will print wall murals like this for you, or you can just write down quotes that speak to you, quotes you can hang on your fridge, bathroom mirror, or bulletin board. Seeing them every day reminds me to keep going. As I said before, I also create inspiration boards with photos that inspire me. You can include a picture of someone with a great body, a dress or bikini you want to fit into, or just healthy foods that you'd like to make staples in your eating routine.

WATCH THE RIGHT MOVIES: I'll be tired and down in the dumps, and Kev will aim the remote at the TV and say, "Watch this . . . ." He'll show me moments from the *Rocky* films or from the movie *Miracle* or even *Warrior*. Recently he had me watch *Searching for Bobby Fischer*. Movies like this always inspire me. Just the other night he cued up one of the final scenes in *Rocky Balboa* in which Rocky says to his son: "*It ain't about how hard you hit. It's about how hard you can get hit and keep moving forward. How much you can take and keep moving forward.*" And I did pick myself up and keep moving forward! As will you!

↓ You can go to *astekwallcovering.com* to design and order a wall like this for yourself! I love the daily reminders.

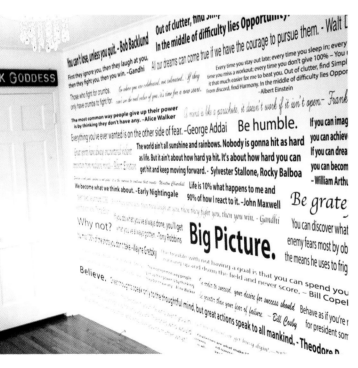

WATCH THE RIGHT TV: I'm pretty obsessed with shows like *South Park* and *Impractical Jokers*. Shows like that make the time fly by while I'm running on the treadmill or doing strength exercises.

PREPARE: I like to lay my workout clothes on the floor next to my bed before I go to sleep. Not only is it a visual reminder that I have a scheduled workout, but it also makes it easy to just slip into my gear and get going. This helps to prevent the "getting ready to go" part of working out from becoming another obstacle.

THE EVERYGIRL'S GUIDE TO DIET AND FITNESS

STAY ON TRACK

To make sticking with exercise even easier, try these tips:

Keep workout gear in the trunk of your car. *I keep a set in mine. If I ever have the urge to work out when I'm away from home, having the clothing on hand makes it easy.*

Change into workout gear at work instead of waiting to change when you get to the gym. *If you don't, there is a chance you could lose the urge to work out and drive home instead.*

Drink coffee on the way to the gym or before working out. *I got this tip from Jillian Michaels. It gives you a quick pick-me-up to get you through.*

When driving to the gym, crank the tunes. *When I drive to the gym, I'm in my workout clothes and listening to my favorite music to get myself pumped up for the workout ahead.*

When on the treadmill, I always tell myself, "Five more minutes and I'll finish." *When the five minutes are over, I'll say, "Hmm, do you think you can make it five minutes more?" Usually, I do. This is how I am able to build up to eventually having runs that last up to forty-five minutes. Once you get through the first fifteen minutes, it gets easier.*

On the treadmill, I walk fast for a solid ten to fifteen minutes *to get my cardio going, then I'll run. If I don't do it this way, the running will never happen.*

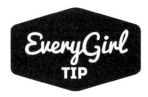

Every Girl TIP

The Nike Training Club app is amazing. Not only does it give you workouts with photos, but also includes instructional videos.

SET REWARDS: Tell yourself that you'll treat yourself to an indulgence, say a massage after every twenty-five workouts. Knowing you've got a goal and a treat coming soon is very motivating!

EMBRACE TECHNOLOGY: The age of social and news media has given us so many options in the physical fitness arena. For example, YouTube is an amazing source for workout videos, but there is so much more. Manufacturers as well as consumers post amazing "how-to" videos on fitness and diet products. This will help you decide if a product is right for you or instruct you on the proper technique. There is also a wide and amazing assortment of tips, tricks, and techniques posted by trainers, experts, as well as nonprofessionals who just want to share information. And when it comes to cooking and making healthy snacks and meals, there are thousands of videos that can give you some tips or even teach you to cook, not to mention the gazillion healthy recipes out there.

I also like Twitter, because I can see what other people are doing for workouts, and that gives me ideas for new moves. Even just reading a tweet from a friend who just did a great workout is helpful. I think: *Well, if she just did that, then I better get out there, too.* It's not so much of a competitive thing as an inspirational thing. It's even better if you can follow someone who is in the process of getting fit whom you can follow in real time.

Here are some great websites and aspirational people to follow:

Stacy Keibler / SKPHILOSOPHY.COM

Perez Hilton / PEREZHILTON.COM/FITPEREZ

Jamie Sherrill / NURSEJAMIE.COM

Giada De Laurentiis / GIADADELAURENTIIS.COM

Bethenny Frankel / BETHENNY.COM

Suzanne Somers / SUZANNESOMERS.COM

Jessica Alba / HONEST.COM

Andrea Orbeck / ANDREAORBECK.COM

Yogi Cameron / YOGICAMERON.COM

Harley Pasternak / HARLEYPASTERNAK.COM

COMPETE: It might not be for everyone, but little bouts of competition can keep you moving forward. Some people like weight-loss contests at work, and I like to identify certain runners ahead of me during a race to see if I can catch up to them. And you know I love my basketball. Some people like to join local rec leagues so they can play the sports they loved in high school. Just injecting a little friendly competition into your exercise routine can be a powerful motivator.

FIND SUCCESS STORIES: Whether you read them in magazines or online by just typing "I lost fifty pounds" into a search engine, you'll find stories about people who have overcome all kinds of obstacles to reach their goals. Many times, seeing what other people have done can help get you out the door. It's also a reminder that success is possible and doable and that you're not alone. You may get some cool tips, too.

I remember reading a *People* magazine article about a poor, single, and courageous mom who lost over a hundred pounds. I put it up on the wall. It inspired me to keep going.

↓ My old size 12 Calvin's

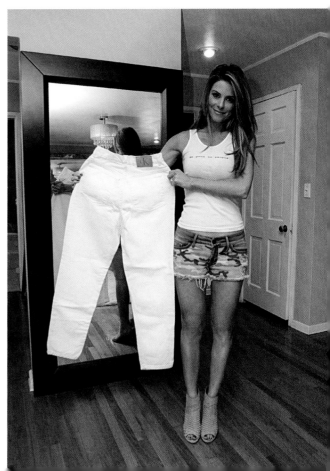

What is your philosophy on weight loss?

I believe in indulging and allowing rather than restricting and de-priving. We need to develop a healthy relationship with food so we can have a little bit of everything. Being "naturally thin" is about treating your diet as a bank account and balancing your good and bad investments.

What is your philosophy on health?

We do the best we can and do what we can when we can. Sleep is the most valuable commodity in the world and will maintain your physical and mental health. I wish I drank more water, and I wish I had the time to exercise regularly. I choose sleep and motherhood first. Those are the healthiest choices for me right now.

What motivates you to stay healthy and active?

You get out of things what you put in, and you feel better when you move. That said, I am in a period of stress and have little time for exercise. I walk when I can and do what I can when I can. I will get back there again.

What's your best advice for someone struggling to lose weight?

You are probably restricting and beating yourself up and bingeing. Use common sense, make small changes, reduce plate size and portion size, and breathe. Never eat out of emotion. You can have a cookie or a piece of pizza. You cannot beat yourself up and binge.

What's one food people should consider subtracting from their diets and one food they should think of adding?

I don't deprive. Add high-volume foods—pureed vegetable soups, dark

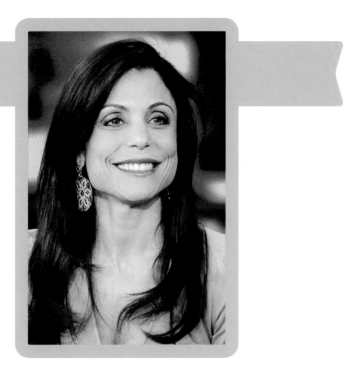

green salads, and green vegetables—but make them taste good.

Q **What do you grab to eat or drink during your day if you need an energy boost?**

Dark chocolate with nuts or a few bites of dessert or black licorice. Sweets in small quantities.

Q **What is your workout schedule?**

I have none. Right now I work out once or twice a week max and just go walking or bike riding. I love to feel good after exercise but don't have time right now. Happiness would be yoga four times a week.

Q **How do you stay in shape?**

Eating is 90 percent of the battle. I eat a variety of foods, I drink Skinnygirl cocktails, and I enjoy without overindulging.

Q **How do you deal with guilt when you've eaten something not in line with your goals or missed a workout?**

Just deal with it.

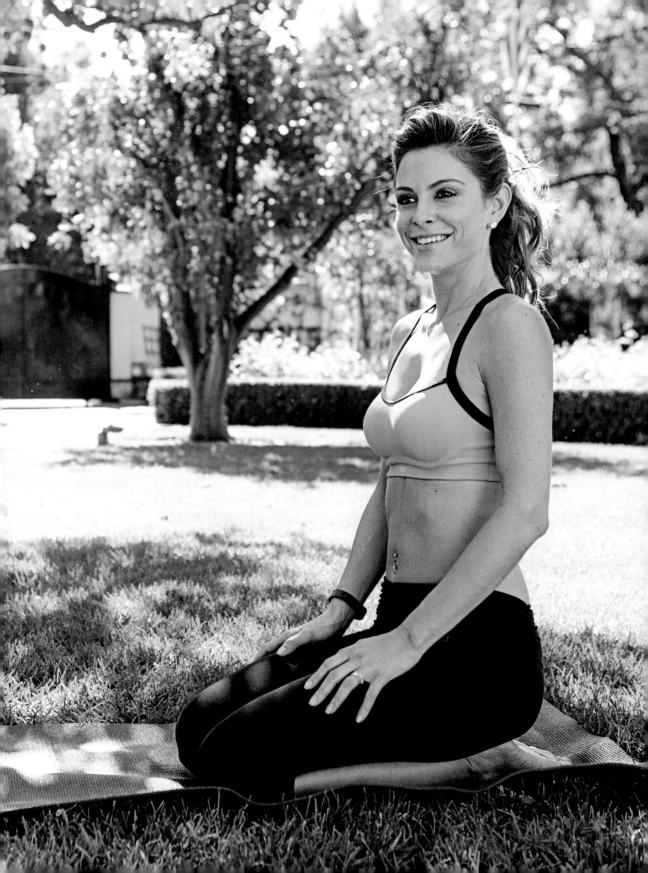

Chapter 12

EveryGirl's Stress-Busting Maintenance Plan

In this chapter, I want to tell you about one of the worst enemies you'll be fighting in your quest to stay fit: stress.

When you are stressed, your body releases a hormone called cortisol. Too much cortisol is the enemy of EveryGirl who is trying to lose weight. First, cortisol triggers appetite. What's worse, it makes you crave quick sources of energy like refined carbs and sugar, and it makes your brain like those foods more than it otherwise would. And if all that wasn't bad enough, cortisol will make you store more fat and will put it right where you don't want it: in your belly.

It's an ugly cycle. You're stressed, so you eat. Eating makes you more stressed, so you eat even more. Clearly, addressing the stress in your life is essential if you want to lose weight and keep it off.

Stress is a big problem in our country, especially for women.

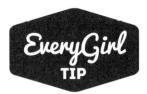

ONE WORKOUT SESSION COULD BE EQUAL TO ONE PROZAC

I know you've heard of the runner's high. It occurs because exercise causes your brain to produce chemicals called endorphins that make you feel good. But you don't have to be a runner. You can get the same effect from any good workout. In fact, a study from the world-famous Cooper Institute in Dallas, Texas, found that people who weren't responding to antidepressant drugs did so much better and had their depression lift once they started exercising. So if you're depressed or just seeking a positive flood of endorphins, here is another good excuse to get a workout in!

I recently came across an interesting report from the American Psychological Association. On a scale of 1 to 10, with 10 being a lot of stress, women on average rated their stress level a 5.3. But one out of every five women said that their stress level was an 8, 9, or a 10! And nearly a third of the women in the study said that they eat to cope with stress. I've certainly had my stress issues (I told you about my rash), and I've been known to give in and reach for all kinds of comfort foods. I try to keep stress in check and deal with it in a healthy way, but it's a constant struggle and one I try to overcome daily.

You obviously can't get rid of all the stress in your life, and really, you wouldn't want to, because *a little* stress is good for you. It's what drives us to grow and move forward. Fortunately, exercise and getting enough sleep, two things I've suggested you do throughout this book, help your body use cortisol so that it isn't as likely to cause all of those nasty side effects. That's why I recommend taking a walk when you have a craving. You burn calories instead of taking them in, but you also squelch that cortisol so that the craving goes away. But there are other ways to calm your life down, and I want to take a little time to discuss them here.

Rage Against Clutter

We've talked about decluttering and organizing your personal spaces. But after you do, you may slip back into bad habits. If you lapse here, chances are you'll lapse in other areas, too, such as your health. Stay vigilant, and don't wait for everything to pile up again. Do a little decluttering each day. You will save yourself time, and it won't feel like such a big job. The benefits are worth the effort. When I first moved to L.A., I thought I'd actually save time if I just threw my clothes on the floor, tossed the mail on the table, and left the

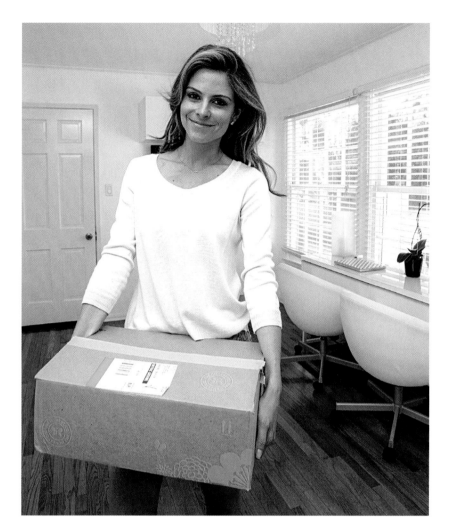

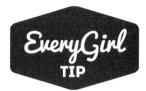
Even though I maintain my clutter-free lifestyle during the year, things do pile up. So when the end of the year rolls around, I do one big purge in which I attack every closet, drawer, and room in the house—including the garage and other storage areas if I can. I toss things out I don't need. I get rid of clothes I never wear. I go through files and dump the nonessentials. If you maintain your space throughout the year, it's not as daunting as it sounds. One of the reasons I love doing it is that it allows me to start the new year strong: fresh, prepared, and ready. I always feel better after I do it. Because I wanted to make this upcoming new year purge even easier, I did a special end-of-summer cleanup and felt like a million bucks after I did. It gave me more free time to enjoy my Christmas break. And you don't need to wait for a new year, either. Spring cleaning, summer solstice, back-to-school time—there's always a turning point in the year when you can make a big sweep.

kitchen a mess. But lazy people really do work the hardest. Besides creating a subconsciously depressing environment for myself, it took me so long to find things I needed—if I ever found them—that I was burning up all my free time. Again, while it may seem like staying organized has very little to do with food and exercise, making sure that you keep your home and work spaces clean and clutter-free will have health benefits that trickle down to all the decisions you make throughout the day.

Stretch Regularly

As we get older, our muscles stiffen, and we lose range of motion. Bending and daily activities (let alone exercise) become harder to do. Even though my dad has great muscle tone, he is definitely more stiff and less mobile than he used to be. The doctors say that this may be partly due to his diabetes, but it's mostly that he didn't stretch enough. Working two jobs and supporting a family, he didn't have time for stretching, and back then, no one really knew how important it was. Stretching helps muscles maintain their youth and elasticity. Just look at the elderly yogis in India and Thailand who are still very flexible and do yoga daily.

A regular stretching program feels good, relieves pains and stress, and lengthens muscles, keeping them spry and youthful. In addition, stretching is believed to reduce the chance of injury as well as increase circulation and energy levels. It also gives you a chance to breathe, slow down, and calm your mind, which helps you control stress. I get my stretching in with yoga, but you don't need to do yoga. Stretch daily if you can—while you watch TV, sit at your desk, or prepare dinner. And it's great to stretch after your muscles are already warm, so do it after a workout or a walk.

Bob Backlund is a WWE professional wrestler and a two-time WWE champion, and he is a testament to the benefits of stretching. Bob has been a friend since I was eighteen, and I recently had the honor of inducting him into the WWE Hall of Fame. Bob is sixty-five years old and is, no exaggeration, in better condition than 99.9 percent of guys in their twenties. Talk about the fifty-year plan in action! He eats fresh fare only and works out every day. Bob is probably the only person in that age group I know who is fitter than my dad. One of the things Bob does to remain on top is stretching,

↓ Made this Bob Backlund T-shirt especially for SummerSlam.

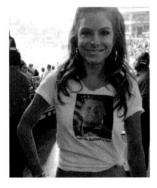

THE EVERYGIRL'S GUIDE TO DIET AND FITNESS

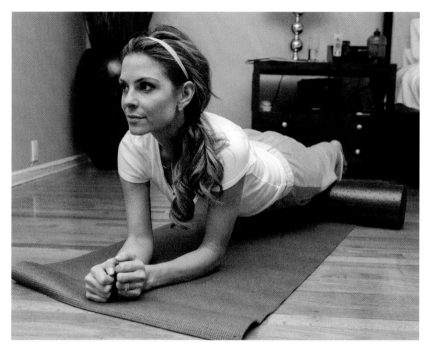

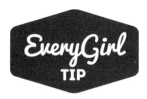
FOAM ROLLERS

A foam roller is a cheap tool I keep under my bed that I can use by myself and that substitutes for a sports massage. By using your own body weight, this cylindrical roller helps you to stretch and work out knots in muscle tissue. It's a must-get!

↑ Lying plank style on the roller, use your upper body to roll up and down against the roller on your quads. Do this on calves and anywhere else you feel would be helpful.

↓ Lie on the foam roller across your shoulder blades, feet shoulder width apart, hands behind head, using your legs to roll your upper back along the roller. Works wonders!

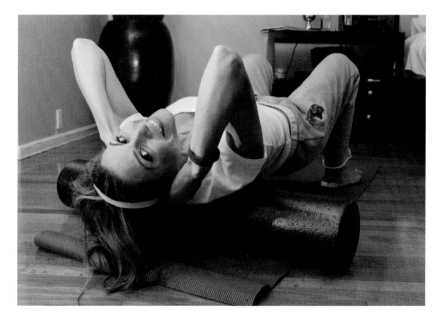

which he does three to five times a day. It's not like Bob is retired. He owns an oil-delivery business, and he even drives the truck himself. Like me, Bob is always moving and always seeking to squeeze fitness into his daily activities and routine. While the oil is pumping, he'll take five minutes to do his stretches. When he is filling up the truck with gas, he stretches. On the phone with clients, he stretches. See how it works?

I'll show you some specific stretching routines in the Appendix, but for now, just try these tips:

➜ Stretch before you get out of bed. That's what I do. I reach down and touch my toes, stretch my back side to side, and so on. Every little bit counts.

➜ Hire a good trainer to teach you stretches to do on your own. Or have him stretch you and your partner and then teach you both how to stretch each other.

➜ Look into taking a tai chi class. This is an "internal martial art" that is often practiced more for its health benefits than for fighting. It's a meditative practice that helps to relieve the body of stress while centering the mind and soul. Though not really considered traditional stretching, the movements involved will help keep muscles limber.

➜ Work on areas that you typically consider tight (like hamstrings), but don't ignore the places where many people store tension, such as the neck and upper back. You can reduce some of that tension by doing light neck stretches at your desk.

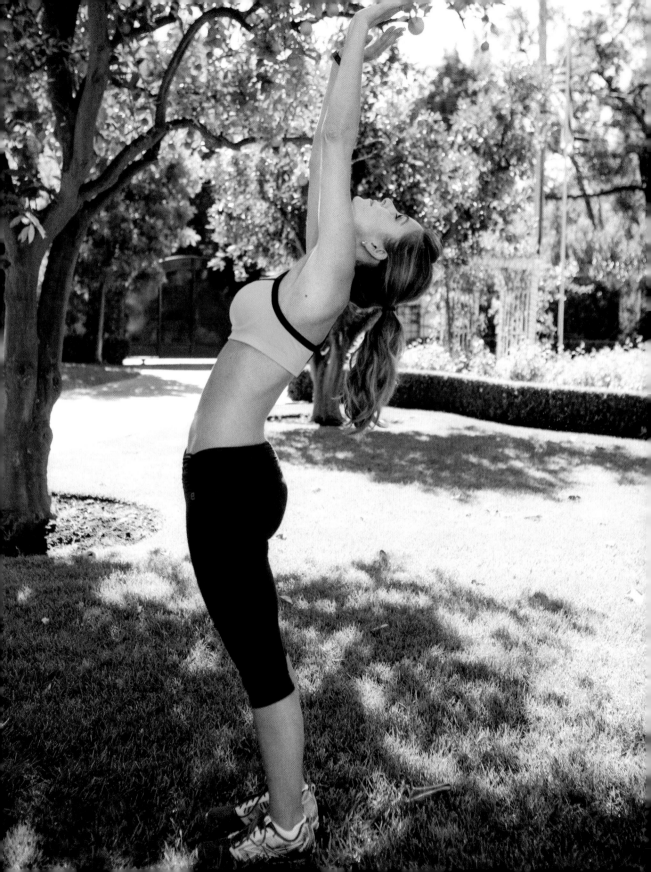

Treat Yourself to Massages

Massages can help relieve soreness and stress and can help flush toxins out of your body. They'll make you feel more flexible and help improve your posture, too. I know some people who like to use massages as rewards—they'll treat themselves to one if they hit a certain exercise or weight-loss goal. There are more and more affordable massage stores popping up in places like the mall, but there are other affordable alternatives.

➜ If you get a good masseur at a spa, ask them if they do house calls. Many like the opportunity for side work. It's more private, convenient, and maybe cheaper, too.

➜ If you're going to spring for a massage, then consider getting a Thai massage. It's usually cheaper in price AND incorporates massage and stretching.

➜ When you are shopping at the mall, hit the gadget stores that have all the massage chairs and devices. Take a load off, sit in the chairs and get yourself a quick, free massage. You may like it so much that you want to buy one; I have a massager that I use on my upper back, and it cost less than fifty dollars.

➜ Brookstone has those amazing Tempur-Pedic slippers. When you come home from work after a long day in heels, there's no better relief for your feet than slipping on a pair.

➜ Rolling a kitchen rolling pin over sore muscles is an excellent way to give yourself or someone else a massage. I've gotten Mom and Dad to do it to one another at the end of every day.

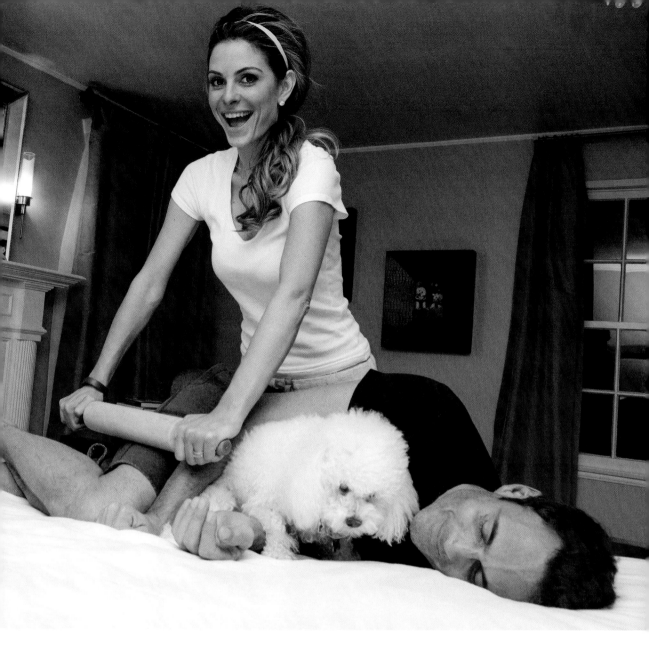

→ Get into a whirlpool. If you don't have one, take a hot bath in Epsom salts after a workout or to end your day. Bed Bath & Beyond has great items like bath pillows, candles, and salts to turn a bath into a rejuvenating spa experience.

↑ You can use a foam roller, but sometimes using a rolling pin is way more fun!

Do you have a favorite saying that keeps you motivated?

> *My father always used to say, "You can only do your own best."
> My mother said, "If your heart is open, it will never stay broken."
> My other mantra is, literally, to "Stop and smell the roses."*

What is your philosophy on weight loss?

> *I think the minute you announce a diet, it's impossible to keep. To
> me weight loss is a new way of looking at food, your relationship
> to food, and the type of food you ingest. So doing a crazy diet
> never works. I weigh myself every day, and I try to stay within six
> pounds of my ideal weight. I know if I lose too much weight, I look
> older. They say you can never look too thin, but you definitely can.*

What is your philosophy on health?

> *I'm a great believer in the combination of Eastern and Western
> medicine. Diagnostically, you can't beat Western medicine, but I do
> believe in listening to my body and knowing what my risk factors
> are genetically and then trying to do the best I can nutritionally.*

What motivates you to stay healthy and active?

> *I was playing Maria Callas in Spain and had a near-death expe-
> rience and needed to be resuscitated. I remember clearly that
> I didn't want to die, and I wanted to go back to my body. From
> that moment I've looked at my body as a car, and if I want to
> drive in that car, I have to make sure it is well maintained. ·*

What do you do to stay in shape?

> *When I'm at home, I work out three times a week at least with a
> trainer, doing cardio on a spin bike, jumping on a Pilates machine,*

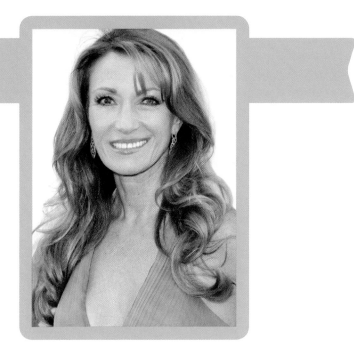

or using a Gyrotonic with light weights. My major motivations with workouts are working on flexibility and weight-bearing exercises for bone health and cardiovascular exercise for the heart. And stomach muscles are really, really important. I've been doing Pilates long before anybody had heard of it. I started in 1976.

Q How do you deal with guilt when you've eaten something you "shouldn't" or miss a workout?

I accept my shortcomings, try to have a sense of humor about it, don't wallow in the past, and decide to do it the next day.

Q You have a great body at the age of sixty-two. What do you credit most for that?

I think a healthy attitude toward food. I am a foodie. I love, love great food, and I suppose I just do everything in moderation, including alcohol, and I never smoke.

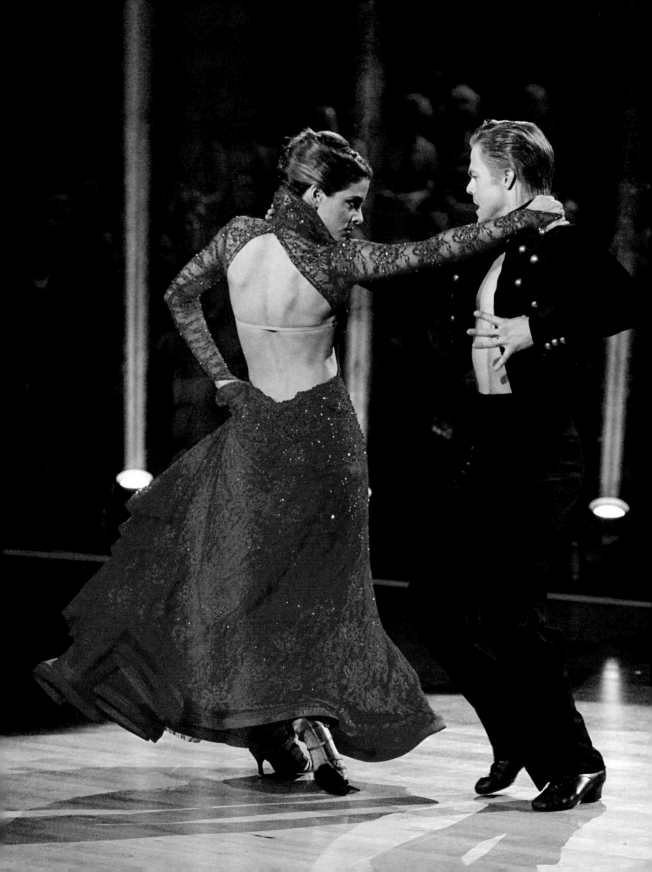

Keep Moving Forward

Of all the tips and strategies I've laid out in this book, the one I hope you remember the most is: Keep moving. Now let me add another layer to that. Keep moving, for sure; but as much as possible, keep moving . . . *forward*. Remember those lines from *Rocky Balboa*? Here they are again: "*It ain't about how hard you hit. It's about how hard you can get hit and keep moving forward. How much you can take and keep moving forward.*" Those words should resonate with everyone. As long as you're inching forward, it doesn't matter how badly you fail, how far you fall short of your goal, or how many punches life gives you. As long as you keep moving forward, even centimeters at a time, you'll be all right.

This principle really hit home for me while standing backstage at *Dancing with the Stars* wearing a red dress and chattering vampire fangs, Derek and I were about to dance the paso doble. I remember saying that the dance, called "Montagues and Capulets," named after Shakespeare's *Romeo and Juliet,* was kind of like our relationship: We love one another, but we may end up killing each other.

I struggled so hard to learn the dance but just couldn't grasp it.

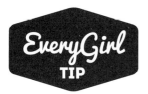

EveryGirl TIP

IF YOU FALL
OFF THE WAGON

I've seen people derail their goals permanently because they slipped back into bad habits. But you can always make a change. As I said, there are days, weekends, or even whole weeks I eat like crap. So what do I do? I catch myself at some point and then go back to healthier ways. You can go back to cleaner eating and being active, or gradually cut back from where you are now. Remember, it's not about being on or off a weight-loss plan. It's about a lifestyle. If you overate or skipped a few workouts, just decide that you will eat healthier at your next meal or that you will exercise at the very next opportunity.

Every practice session we had, I messed up one part of the step or another. The competition on the show had gotten more intense and now, standing backstage seconds before the dance, I was thinking about how I originally didn't want to do the show. I had never been any kind of dancer. "Why did I allow myself to do this?!" Then I started feeling even worse for poor Derek. In the past, some of Derek's other partners *had* been dancers. They must have been so much easier to train, and none of them embarrassed him, as I feared I was about to. As I said, my parents and Kev were in the crowd, too. I didn't want them to see me make a fool of myself. I was nervous, anxious, and terrified.

And then the music cued and we took to the stage. I don't remember much. I just let myself go and followed Derek's lead—until the end. At that point, I opened my mouth, displayed my fangs and "bit" Derek in the neck, wiped his fake blood from my mouth, and stood in a silence that seemed to last an eternity. And then . . . the standing ovation from the crowd. It still didn't hit me how well we had done until I saw Derek. I could tell from his look that he was altogether relieved, proud, and stunned. And then the judges confirmed it.

Carrie Ann: "That was amazing. You were so on fire."

Len: "Sharp as a razor. Crisp as a Pringle. And more tension than my grandmother's knicker elastic. You lived it, and I loved it. Fantastic."

Bruno: "The way you two played together was absolutely spell-binding."

When we received all 10s, the first perfect dance of the season, I couldn't believe it. I think Derek and I even chest-bumped after we saw the scores! But the bigger point isn't that we performed well. (I didn't go on to win the competition and, incidentally, I didn't win the Miss Massachusetts USA beauty pageant back in 2000, either.) Even more important than winning that night, those experiences *moved me forward*. Just as the pageant inspired me to lose the extra weight I had been carrying, being on *Dancing with the Stars* helped me get fitter and opened my eyes to so many things. It was one of the most amazing experiences of my life—and I almost didn't experience it. Had I not opted to put my fears aside and step out of my comfort zone, I wouldn't have experienced any of it. Had I not kept my mind in the state of possibility, had I not been open to always improving myself, it never would have happened. With *Dancing with the Stars,* I broke bones and I didn't win but none of that mattered because I moved forward.

The Most Important Lesson

Life will *always* get in the way at some point, knocking you down, making it hard for you to maintain healthy behavior. Or maybe you'll get complacent, happy with what you've accomplished and then overindulge. Guess what? I experience all of the above to this very day, so welcome to the club. All we can do is brush off and try again. I told you, if you're not growing, you're dying, but if you're not trying, you're doing the same.

One Last Story

Inducting my old friend, professional wrestler and diet and fitness inspiration Bob Backlund into the WWE Hall of Fame was an honor. It was also one of the most inspirational experiences of my life, even though this time I didn't receive a standing ovation. On the contrary, I was booed by *all* of Madison Square Garden.

I met Bob when I met Kev, working on Kev's first movie. I was just an eighteen-year-old film student, and I remembered when my dad and I would watch him wrestle on TV, so I was starstruck.

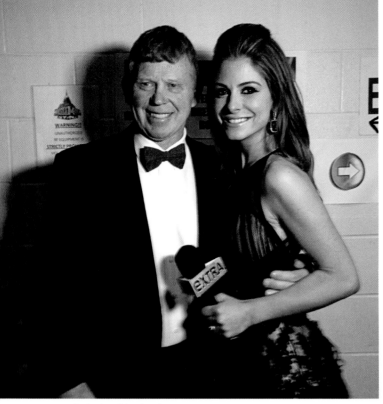

↑ My dear friend and champion Mr. Bob Buckland.

Bob was so sweet to everyone on the set, and we became good friends. He was always supportive of Kev and me, including sitting in the front row at that 2000 Miss Massachusetts USA beauty pageant.

Like Jack LaLanne and my dad, Bob, as I said, is a poster child for the fifty-year plan, working out every day and eating a healthy diet. Yet his life was not without disappointment and heartache. When Hulk Hogan replaced him as champion in the mid-1980s, the powers that be asked Bob to become a villain—a "heel" as they call it. But Bob didn't want to do that. Back then, wrestling was not yet considered sports entertainment. Bob was working with needy children who looked up to him. Turning heel would let them down. On top of that, this was a time when steroids and drugs were beginning to creep into wrestling, and Bob wanted nothing to do with that. He left wrestling and went from performing in stadiums in front of tens of thousands of roaring fans to working construction and doing odd jobs. I don't know if he would admit it, and I hope he's not mad that I'm saying it, but I think deep down he was heartbroken, and understandably so. His kindness, decency, and moral compass had cost him his dream and career. But God bless Bob, because he kept trying. Many people made fun of him, and a lot of people thought he was crazy, but through his forties, fifties, and way beyond, he kept eating right and working out, hoping, I believe, to return to wrestling one day.

I'm compressing Bob's inspirational story, because it's better for him to tell it one day, as I hope he will. But the long and short of it is that Bob not only made it back, he made it back in the biggest way: being inducted into the WWE Hall of Fame. I was so honored when Bob asked me to induct him. It was totally a full circle. He supported me when I was a teen, and now I would get the chance to do the same for him. I prepared a long speech about

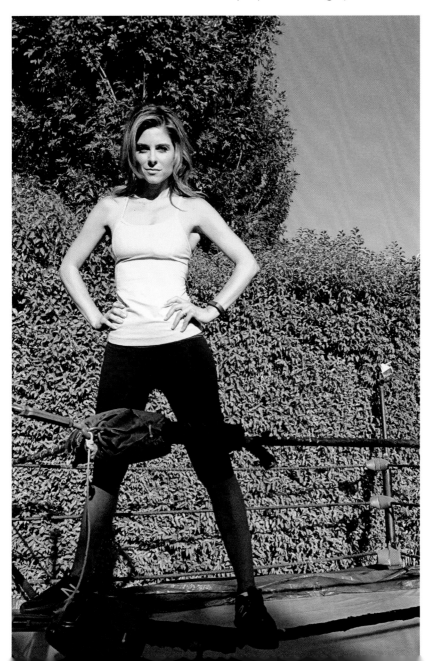

his many accomplishments. I was so excited to tell the world what I already knew: Bob is more than a champion, he is a real-life hero. But the wrestling fans didn't take kindly to a "celebrity" inducting a wrestler. They booed me throughout the entire speech. Eventually, the jeers grew so loud that you couldn't even hear what I was saying. I finished the speech and handed the microphone to Bob and then went backstage, holding back my tears. Stephanie McMahon, one of the owners of WWE, is a dear friend. Her dad, Vince, who rarely grants interviews these days, spoke on my behalf on *Dancing with the Stars* and said the most amazing things about me, which was a gesture I'll never forget. Stephanie's husband, Paul Levesque, known as "Hunter" or "Triple H," has been equally supportive and helped me to achieve my dream to wrestle. After I was booed off the stage, Steph put her hands on my shoulders and assured me that everything was fine. I was humiliated, but the worst of it was that I felt as if I had totally let Steph, Vince, Hunter, and especially Bob down. I ruined a moment that he had worked decades for. He deserved to have everyone in that audience hear about all the

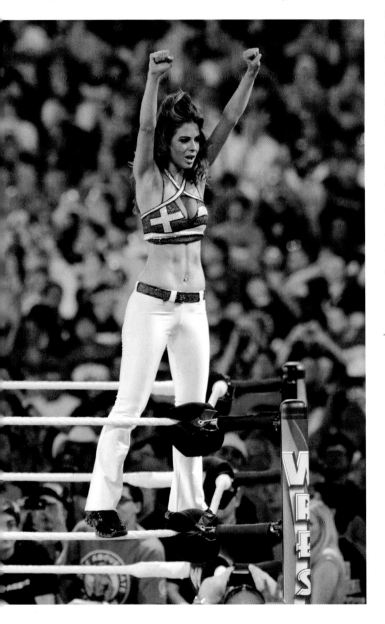

↓ Amazing memory: Seventy thousand screaming fans.... Thank you Derek Hough for the gorgeous picture you took.".

THE EVERYGIRL'S GUIDE TO DIET AND FITNESS

amazing accomplishments he had attained over the years. And then like so many things, what I thought was one of the worst experiences in my life turned into one of the best—or at least one of the most enlightening.

After Stephanie consoled me, Kev pulled me to one of the TV monitors and said, "Honey, it's fine." I said, "It's *not* fine." Then he said reassuringly, "Shhh, just watch." On the screen was Bob, who had by now silenced the entire garden with his words. Finishing his speech, he screamed a phrase that will inspire me for the rest of my life: "You never lose unless you quit!"

But Bob wasn't done. Not by a freaking long shot. Exiting, he screamed the next line even louder and with a huge grin: "Tonight I'm going to enjoy myself!" For good measure, he then added, " . . . and I'm going to keep fighting!"

It didn't matter who was booing me or making fun of him, Bob was damn well going to enjoy himself. And regardless of what anyone said or did, he was going to keep fighting. And that's it, ladies. When it comes to weight loss, fitness, and any part of your life's journey: You never lose unless you quit. And no matter what anyone says about you, what grand, different, or odd challenges you take on, how foolish you may look while trying or how big you may fail, you just enjoy yourself and you keep fighting!

I'm rooting for all of you and hope the information in this book helps you as much as it helped me. If you are having a hard time in your weight loss and health journey or have any questions, you can always ask me on Twitter—just find me at @MariaMenounos. Many women already do, and I love it. I also love how much I learn from you all as well. If you have tips, tricks, and helpful information on diet, health, and fitness, be sure to tweet them as well. It's how we all keep growing and moving forward.

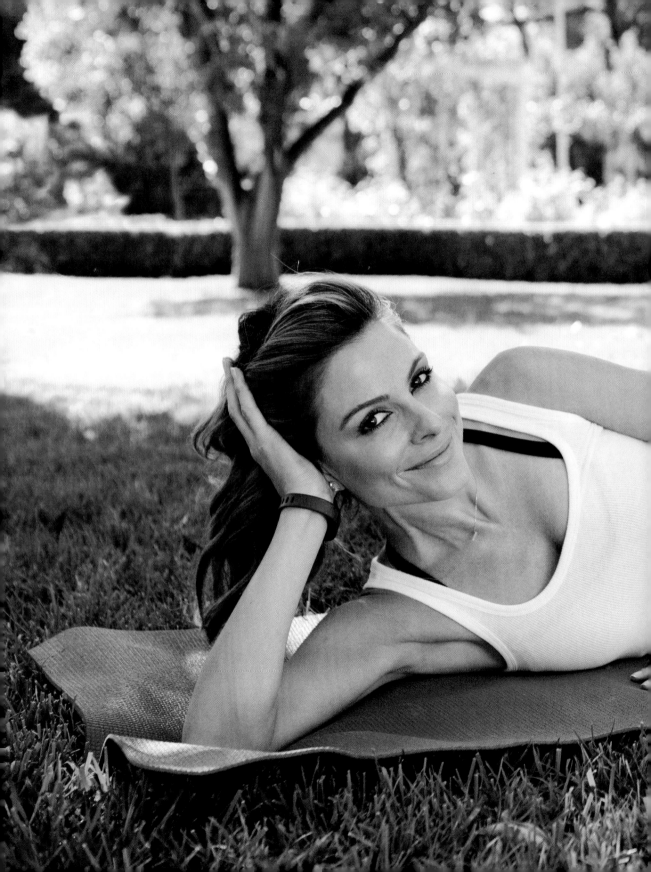

The EveryGirl Workouts

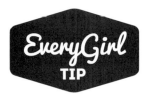

TO TONE ABS

While engaging in all exercises make a conscious effort to tighten your abs. This anytime, anywhere move helps to further strengthen and tone your core. I tighten my abs during all my exercises. Every extra bit helps.

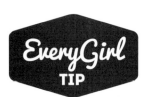

Take photos of these routines with your camera phone so you can use them anywhere.

Throughout this book, I've tried to give you many different ideas for how to train and how to incorporate both formal and informal workouts into your life. And the reality is that there are almost as many different kinds and styles of training as there are people. Some like classes, some like to go solo, some like lifting, some like cardio. And you know my bottom line: As long as you keep moving and integrate fitness into your life, you're going to be okay. I did, however, want to give you some more structured plans for working out. Many of these are strength-based (that is, they use some kind of resistance, whether it's bands, body weight, dumbbells, or machines) to help work your muscles and build your strength, which will get you toned and help you burn fat more effectively. I find that these types of workouts don't just make me feel and look better in an outward kind of way, they also help with core strength, posture, and confidence—which are important for all of us as we move through life. So go ahead and give any or all of them a try. And mix and match moves if you like. The routines are designed to work the three main parts of your physique: upper body, lower body, and core, for total-body balance.

The Guidelines

I don't want to force you into a set routine—for instance, saying that you have to do a certain number of workouts for a certain number of days for a certain number of minutes. How you exercise is less important than whether or not you do it. That said, there are some basic guidelines that I like to use, and you can follow them if you are a need-a-routine kind of woman.

➔ For any cardio exercise (that is, any aerobic-type work), it's okay to do it as often as you like and as much as your schedule can stand. It's great for maintaining your heart, burning calories, and keeping your energy levels up. But pay attention to your body, and if you start to feel tweaks in your joints or elsewhere, make sure you mix in some different types of exercise—swim or bike if you're a runner, for example.

→ For strength routines (that is, any workout that involves you pushing or pulling some kind of weight, whether it's a dumbbell, bands, or even your own body weight), it's best to wait at least forty-eight hours between workouts. That allows your muscles to repair themselves—and that's where the real benefits happen! So a general guideline is to not do strength workouts more than three times a week. However, you can alternate upper- and lower-body moves every other day, if you prefer.

→ If this is your first foray into strength training, then you may not be familiar with some of the terms, like *sets* and *reps*. *Rep* is short for "repetitions." Each time you do a movement, that's a rep—so one push-up, for example, is one rep. When you do 10 push-ups in a row without stopping, those 10 reps make up a "set." So you'll see directions that give you a particular number of reps and sets. Those are adjustable based on your time, ability, and other factors. But the recommendations here are some good starting points.

→ I also love to mix things up, so don't think that just because I have a certain routine listed here, it's the only way to do it. I like to mix and match, substitute different exercises, or create my own workouts based on different ideas. So if you see elements from a couple of different workouts that you like, feel free to create your own. Workouts are a lot like recipes—sometimes you have to experiment and add your own flavors to make what tastes best to you.

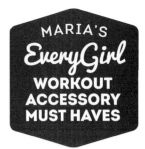

MARIA'S EveryGirl WORKOUT ACCESSORY MUST HAVES

Resistance Bands
Dumbbell/Barbell
Yoga Mat
Medicine Ball

EveryGirl Seven Essential Stretches

I like to stay as flexible as I can—it helped tremendously as I was learning new dances. But I also like it because it helps me feel better, especially when I'm always on the move or have to be stuck sitting a lot. Best of all, they're easy enough to do when you're winding down from a long day or just need something gentle to get you going. Here are some of my favorites that I like to use to keep loose.

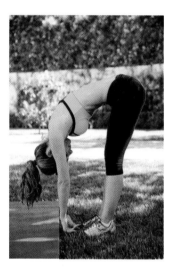

Touch Your Toes/ Hamstring Stretch

With knees straight but not locked, bend at the hips to feel elongation of the hamstrings. Keep your neck relaxed and place your hands on the ground. Hold for 5 breaths.

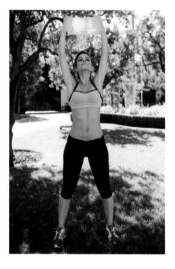

Chest Stretch with Band

Anchor your thumbs or hands in the band and lift your hands above your head. Arch your back and lift your chin, reaching your arms straight behind you. Hold for 5 breaths.

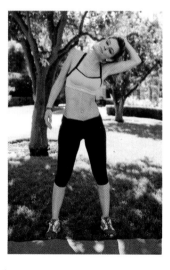

Neck Roll

Slowly roll your neck in circular motions, making sure to go in both directions. After 10 repetitions in each direction, bend your neck to one side and gently pull your head down with your hand for a nice, deep stretch. And then repeat on the other side.

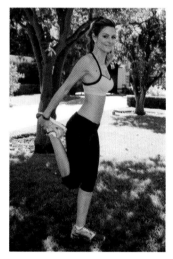

Quad Stretch

Standing upright, bend one knee and hold the heel of that foot against your glute. Hold for 5 breaths.

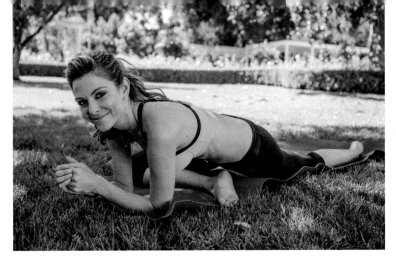

Pigeon Stretch

This stretch really helps loosen up tight hips, as it helps elongate your hip flexors as well as the muscles in your butt. It's actually not as hard as it looks. You start by doing a butterfly stretch with your legs in front of you, then simply lean to one side so that you can slide the opposite leg behind your body. Then lean forward to feel the stretch throughout your hips and butt.

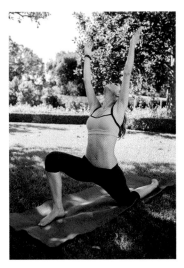

The Psoas Stretch

If you do a lot of sitting, there's a good chance that a small muscle deep within your back and hips (called the psoas) can get very tight—and become the source of back pain. So it's important that you keep that muscle flexible. Here's what you do: Kneel on the floor, keeping your back straight. Now place your right foot on the floor in front of you—this will look a bit like a lunge, but your right foot and left knee will be on the ground. From this position, tilt your tailbone forward a bit and lean your upper body gently back. This will open up the psoas. Repeat with the other leg in front. (You're welcome.)

The Bob Backlund Stretch

I learned this stretch from my friend Bob Backlund, a two-time WWE World Champion. He swore it kept him limber over a career that lasted thirty-plus years. Standing straight with your hands on your hips, lean back. Look up to the sky, hold, relax, and breathe. Stand straight again with hands on your hips, and then bend to one side. Hold, relax, and breathe. Repeat on the other side. Hold, relax, and breathe. Now bend forward, stretch your arms down so the palms of your hands are parallel to the ground. (You may not be able to touch the ground with your palms; do the best you can, but just keep your palms parallel to the ground.)

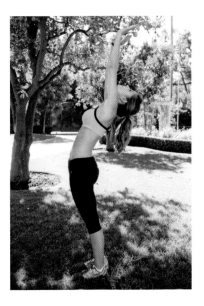

At-Your-Desk Workout

> Depending on your setup, you may want to think about bringing in a light pair of dumbbells to the office. There may be tasks you can do without your hands (say, while you are reading or listening in on a conference call) where you can squeeze in a few moves. Or are you heading out to a work lunch? Do a 5-minute routine before you pack up and go—it'll give you a muscle boost, and it might have the great side effect of discouraging you from eating too much bad stuff at your meal!

OPTION 1 Stretches

Sitting at your desk for long periods of time can tighten your hips, shorten your hamstrings, and push your shoulders forward, leading to back pain and poor posture. Choose any four or five of these stretches and switch them up throughout your day and week.

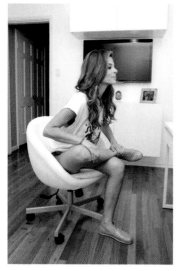

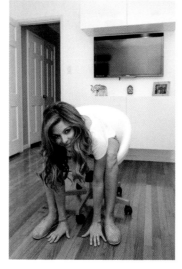

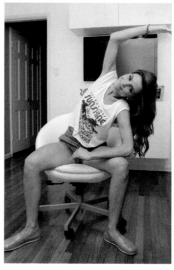

Seated Glute Stretch

With your back straight and one ankle over the opposite knee, bend forward at your hips while pressing the bent knee down to stretch the glute. Hold for 15 seconds per side.

Lumbar Stretch

With your knees apart, bend your body until your hands are on the floor, allowing gravity to stretch your spine. Hold for 5 breaths as you deepen the stretch.

QL Stretch

This is for the muscles that connect your ribs to your hips, which can shorten when you sit for long periods of time.

Leaning to one side with your elbow on your knee, reach the other hand over your head, creating space between the ribs and hips. Hold for 3 breaths. Then repeat on the other side.

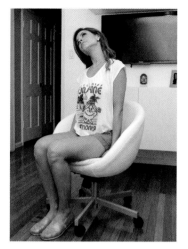

Neck Stretch

Sitting on your hands (palms facing up), tilt one ear to your shoulder while slightly lifting your chin. Maintain the anchor of the opposite hand under your butt. Hold for 5 breaths.

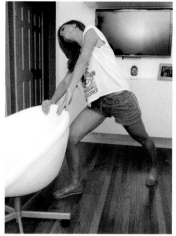

Psoas Stretch

Using the back of the chair for balance and stability, stagger your stance with one foot in front of the other. Lean your body over your front leg, anchoring the back heel into the ground. Hold for 5 breaths.

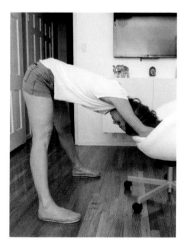

Pec Stretch

Stand with your feet slightly wider than shoulder-width apart and toes forward. Bend your body over a chair with your elbows on the seat and your head below your shoulders. Hold for 5 breaths.

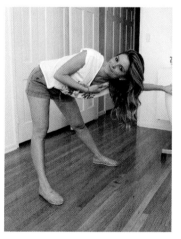

Low-Back Lap Stretch

Using the back of a chair, extend one arm straight with your hand grasping the top of the chair. Hinge the hips over until you feel a stretch in the chest muscles, turning your head away from the extended hand. Hold for 3 breaths.

EASY YOGA MOVES

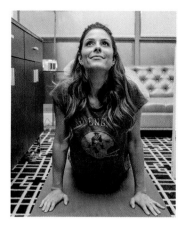

UPWARD DOG OR COBRA

Lying facedown on the mat with your ankles and knees together, legs straight, and chin tucked in, rise up onto your elbows while stretching your abs and slowly transition onto your hands. Draw your shoulders down and back. Hold for 5 breaths.

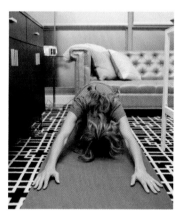

CHILD'S POSE

Starting on your hands and knees, inch your hands forward until your arms are straight and push your butt back so that it is resting on your heels. Relax your spine and hold for 5 breaths.

At-Your-Desk Workout

OPTION 2 Bands, Bars, and Dumbbells

If you have the space and room for a light set of dumbbells, a resistance band, or even a barbell, you can bang out a routine while on a conference call or during a break. Repeat the moves so that you do the entire circuit two or three times.

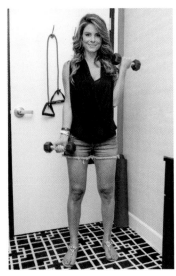

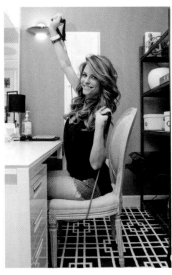

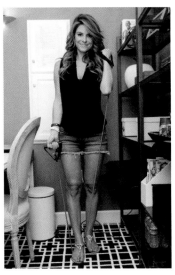

Standing Dumbbell Curl

Stand with your feet shoulder-width apart and in an upright posture holding 5- to 7.5-lb. dumbbells. Hold your elbows at your ribs and alternate bending your elbows, reaching your palms to your shoulders, but don't let your upper arms drift forward. Repeat for a minimum of 40 reps.

TARGET ZONE BICEPS

BONUS ZONE BACK

Overhead Press with Resistance Band

Sit upright on a chair and bend your knees at a 90-degree angle. Place a resistance band under the seat of the chair, grasp an end in each hand, and sit with your chest upright and your hands at shoulder level. Alternately press each hand overhead, drawing one arm back down as you raise the other up. Do 12 reps for each arm.

TARGET ZONE SHOULDERS

BONUS ZONES ABS AND BACK

Standing Biceps Curl with Resistance Band

Stand upright with one foot anchoring the center of the band. Holding the handles with your arms at your sides, alternate bending and straightening your left and your right elbow, bringing the handle of the band up to your shoulder. Do 12 reps for each arm.

TARGET ZONE BICEPS

BONUS ZONE UPPER BACK

288

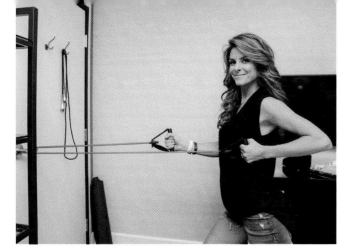

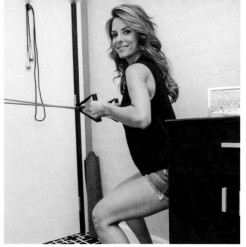

Standing Alternating Row with Resistance Band

Anchor the band around a fixed surface. Standing upright, walk back until your arms are straight with a little tension in the band. Row your elbows back, alternating right and left. Do 30 reps total.

TARGET ZONE BACK

BONUS ZONE BICEPS

Squat with Resistance Band

Stand with your feet on the middle of the band and hold an end in each hand at shoulder level. Bend your hips back and squat down as low as you can while keeping the natural arch in your lower back. Squeeze your glutes as you come back up, pushing through your heels. Do 20 reps.

TARGET ZONE THIGHS

BONUS ZONE BUTT

OPTIONAL

ADD A BARBELL

Barbells may seem clunky, but if you've got room in your office, bring in one, or a Body Bar (as pictured), and throw it in with your other workout routines. It's a great way to add resistance and good for strength training and conditioning.

Barbell Squat

Using a sofa or chair to help you judge the depth of your squats, place the barbell across the backs of your shoulders—not your neck—holding it with your hands about shoulder-width apart. Stand with the sofa or chair close behind you, feet shoulder-width apart and toes pointing slightly outward. Keep your chest up and bend the hips back to squat down until you just barely touch the seat, then drive through your heels to come back up. Repeat 20 times.

TARGET ZONE THIGHS

BONUS ZONE BUTT

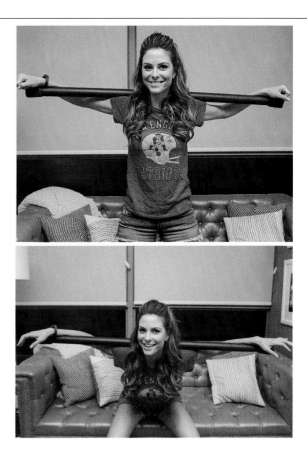

At-Your-Desk Workout

OPTION 3 Hand Weights and Body Weight

Many people don't realize that you can bring the "gym" with you to work and also make it work for you at your own home. Below is a mix of great exercises. Choose any five to make a circuit. Repeat the circuit two or three times.

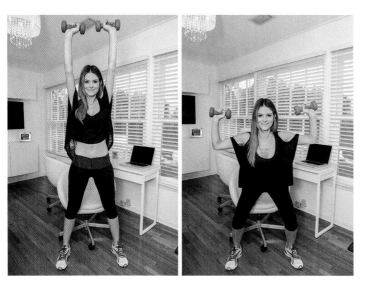

Overhead Press with Squat

Stand with your feet shoulder-width apart with 3- to 5-lb. hand weights over your head.

Lower your hips until your butt almost touches the chair while simultaneously lowering the weights to shoulder level. Return to the start position while pressing the weights overhead. Repeat 20 times.

TARGET ZONES LEGS, QUADS, AND SHOULDERS

BONUS ZONE HEART

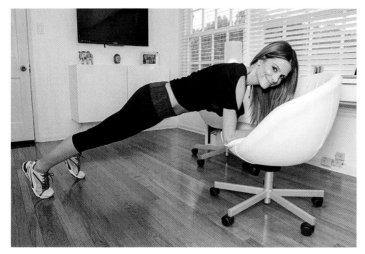

Chair Plank

Bend your elbows 90 degrees and rest your forearms on the seat of a chair. Brace your abs and hold your body in a straight line Your butt should be at the same level as or slightly higher than the shoulders. Aim to hold for at least 30 seconds and gradually work up to a full minute over time.

TARGET ZONE ABS

BONUS ZONE LOWER BACK

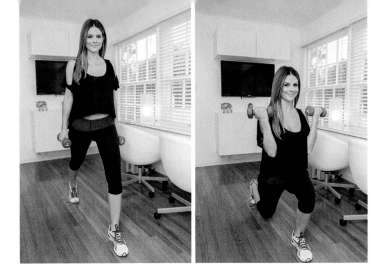

Standing Lunge with Bicep Curl

Get in a split-squat stance with your weight on your front leg, arms at your sides with a 5-lb. (or heavier) dumbbell in each hand.

Lower your leg until the back knee is nearly touching the floor and curl your biceps at the same time. Return to start position and do 10-15 reps. Switch leading legs and repeat.

TARGET ZONES THIGHS AND BICEPS

BONUS ZONE BUTT

Seated Rotator Cuff

Sit with a straight back, holding 5-lb. (or heavier) hand weights, tuck your elbows to your sides and hold your hands out front.

Keeping your elbows tucked to your sides, rotate your hands as far back as you can without letting your elbows leave your sides. Lift your chest as you rotate and return to the start position for 20 repetitions.

TARGET ZONE ROTATOR CUFF

BONUS ZONE UPPER BACK

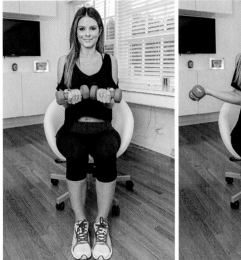
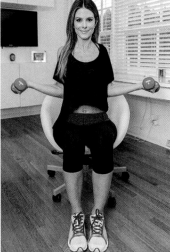

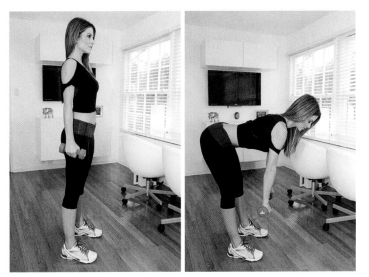

Deadlift

Stand upright with your feet between hip- and shoulder-width apart, knees unlocked, and your back slightly arched with your arms at your sides holding 5-lb. (or heavier) hand weights.

Bend your hips back, lowering your torso until you feel a stretch in your hamstrings. Squeeze your glutes as you return to the starting position. Repeat 12 times.

TARGET ZONE HAMSTRINGS

BONUS ZONE LOWER BACK

WORKOUT CONTINUED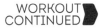

At-Your-Desk Workout

OPTION 3 *(continued from previous page)*

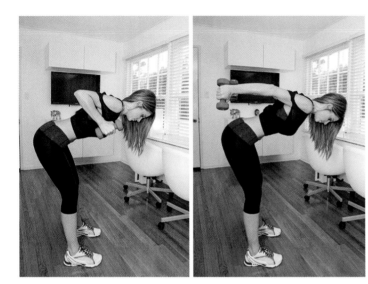

Bent-Over Triceps Press

Bend over at the hips, maintaining a stiff back. With your elbows at your sides, hold 5-lb. hand weights straight down from the elbow.

Keeping your elbows at your sides, use your triceps to straighten your arms and then return to start position. Do 20 reps.

TARGET ZONE TRICEPS

BONUS ZONE BACK

Bent-Over Row

Bending over between a 45- and 90-degree angle, hold two 5-lb. hand weights in front of your knees.

Row both arms as far back as you can and then return to the start position. Repeat 20 times.

TARGET ZONE UPPER BACK

BONUS ZONE LOWER BACK

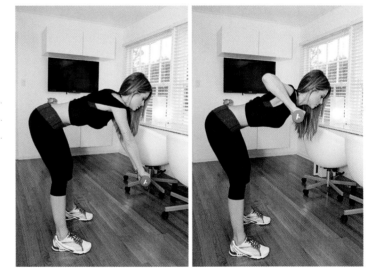

292

First-Position Plié Squat

Using the back of a chair for balance, hold your heels together in a first-position ballet stance, rising up on your toes.

Lower your heels and hips, allowing your knees to move outward as your tailbone drops a few inches into the plié. As you lift to the start position, squeeze your inner thighs together. Repeat 20 times.

TARGET ZONE INNER THIGHS

BONUS ZONE CALVES

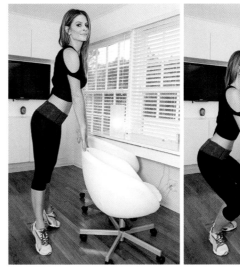
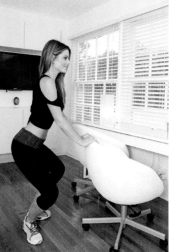

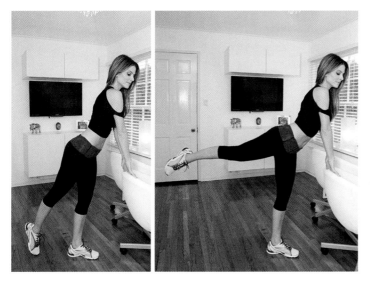

Standing Glute Abduction

Using the back of the chair for balance, stand upright and extend one of your legs behind you, straight and rotated outward slightly. Using your glute, lift your leg as high as you can without arching your back. Hold for a second at the top, squeezing the glute.

Return the leg slowly to the start position, fighting gravity as you return. Repeat each leg a minimum of 20 times.

TARGET ZONE BUTT

BONUS ZONE LOWER BACK

The Bad-Ass Bedside Workout

So you're the kind of woman who can get out of bed and face the day right away? One who don't need no stinkin' java? I love it. But maybe you don't have enough time to squeeze in a full workout before work or family demands your attention. If that's the case, then try this advanced series of moves that will get your muscles all fired up. Repeat this circuit two or three times.

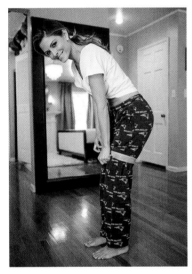

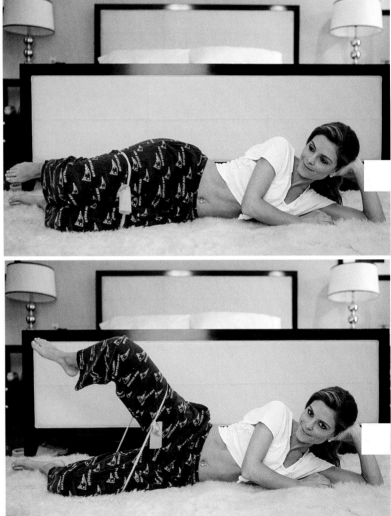

Mermaid

Tie a resistance band around your quads just above the knees.

Lie down on a bed on your side with one knee stacked on the other. Stack your feet as well.

Keep your heels together and lift your top leg away from the bottom one against the resistance of the band. Complete 20 reps on each side.

TARGET ZONE BUTT

BONUS ZONE ABS

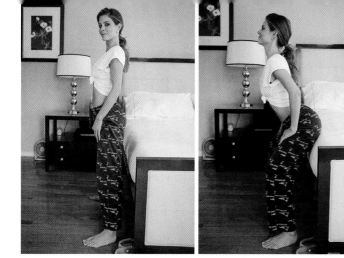

Bed Squat

Stand facing at least 5 inches away from your bed, feet shoulder-width apart, with an upright posture.

Using your quads and glutes, squat until you lightly touch the top of the mattress. Return to start position. Complete 25 reps.

TARGET ZONE THIGHS

BONUS ZONE BUTT

Pistol Squat

Sit close to the edge of the bed, arms out in front of you for balance, one foot raised slightly off the floor.

Rise off the bed until fully upright, pulling the elevated knee into your chest as you stand. Complete 10 repetitions on each leg.

TARGET ZONE THIGHS

BONUS ZONE CORE

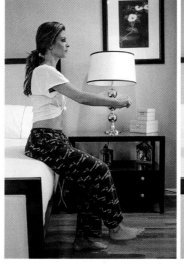

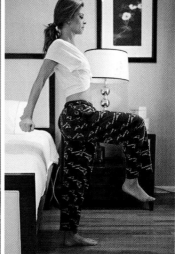

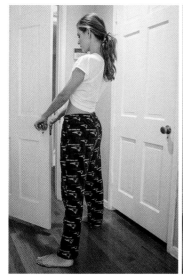

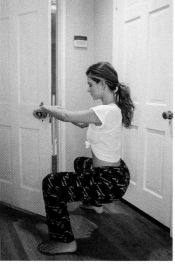

Door Squat

Open a door and stand facing it so it's perpendicular to your body. Stand upright with your feet shoulder-width apart, and grasp a doorknob in each hand. Point your knees slightly out and lean back as if you are waterskiing.

Bend your hips back, maintaining the weight on your heels, and lower your body as far as you can. Return to start position. Repeat for 20 repetitions.

TARGET ZONE THIGHS

BONUS ZONE BACK

WORKOUT CONTINUED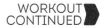

The Bad-Ass Bedside Workout
(continued from previous page)

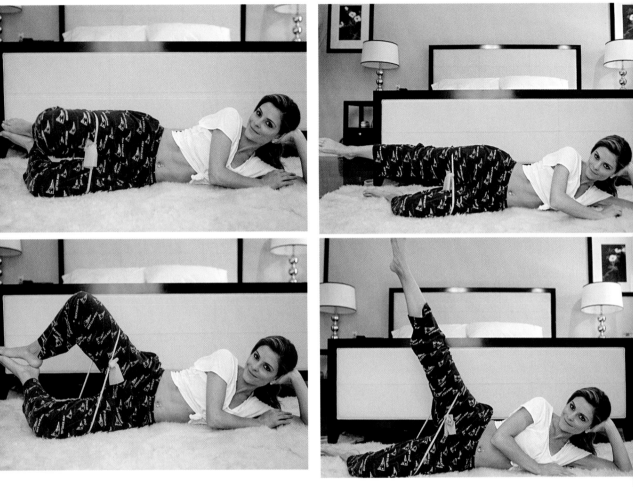

Clams

Set up as you did for the mermaids, with a tied resistance band and knees bent 90 degrees. Your knees and ankles should be stacked on top of each other.

Rotate your top knee away from the bottom one against the resistance of the band. Complete 20 reps on each leg.

TARGET ZONE BUTT

BONUS ZONE ABS

Lateral Leg Lift

With your floor leg bent for stability and balance, straighten your top leg and turn your toe and knee slightly outward.

Raise your straight leg up against the resistance band as high as you can without losing balance. Return to start position. Complete 20 reps on each leg.

TARGET ZONE BUTT

BONUS ZONE HIP FLEXORS

Original EveryGirl Workout (Debbie's)

Growing up, my cousin hired local athlete and trainer Debbie Maida to help me prepare for a pageant. Her workout circuit was the real original EveryGirl workout. I followed it for six months getting ready for the pageant, and I lost 20 pounds. I always aimed to do the most I could every single day—not just two or three days a week. Along with it I did the elliptical. I could do only five minutes on the elliptical to start, but by the end I was doing forty-five minutes a day about three times a week. I aim to complete three full sets of this circuit.

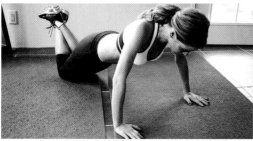

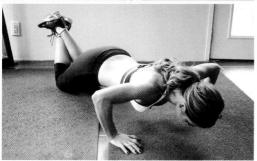

Push-up

With your hands under your shoulders and knees on the ground—you can do toes on the ground, too!—keep your back flat and your butt down.

Lower your frame so that your chest is nearly touching the floor. Complete 10 reps.

TARGET ZONE CHEST

BONUS ZONE TRICEPS

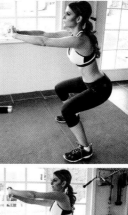

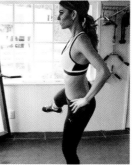

Squat and Side Leg Lift

With your hands out in front of you and feet slightly wider than shoulder-width apart, squat down so that your thighs are parallel to the ground. Concentrate on keeping your butt back.

As you rise back up, extend your left leg out to the side, balancing on one foot. Concentrate on keeping your core tight and look straight ahead to keep your balance.

Squat down again (using two feet), then rise up again, this time lifting your right leg. Complete 10 reps.

TARGET ZONE BUTT

BONUS ZONE CORE

WORKOUT CONTINUED
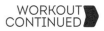

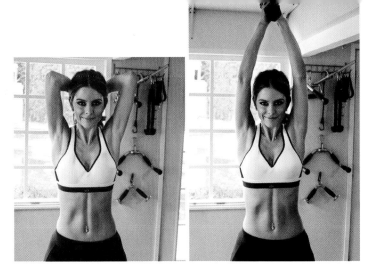

Overhead Triceps Extension

Stand straight and hold a light dumbbell with both hands behind your head. Keep your upper arms perpendicular to the floor.

Without moving the position of your upper arms, extend your elbows to raise the weights up to the ceiling, then lower again. This will really tighten your arms up and lend sleek and strong definition to the backs of your arms. Complete 15 reps.

TARGET ZONE **TRICEPS**

BONUS ZONE **SHOULDERS**

Low Squat Plié

Stand with your feet slightly wider than shoulder-width apart and point your toes out at 45-degree angles.

Squat down, not moving the position of your toes and keeping your butt back. Keep your hands on your hips throughout the movement. Complete 20 reps.

TARGET ZONE **THIGHS**

BONUS ZONE **CALVES**

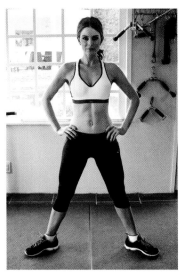

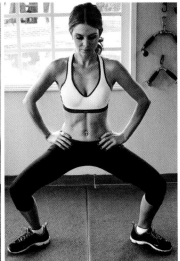

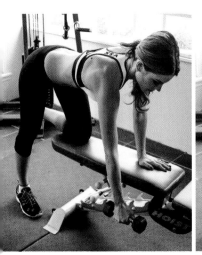

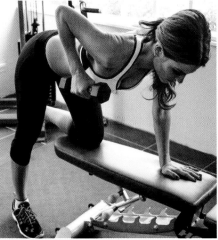

One-Arm Row

I love this one for helping make my back look—and be!—strong. Put your left knee on a bench and keep your right foot on the ground. Hold a dumbbell with your right hand and let your arm hang so that it's perpendicular to your back (which you need to keep level) and the floor.

Without moving your back, pull the weight straight up so that the dumbbell comes to your ribs. Complete 12 reps on each side.

TARGET ZONE **BACK**

BONUS ZONE **BICEPS**

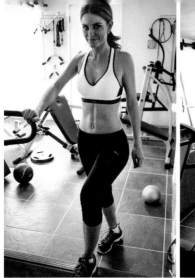
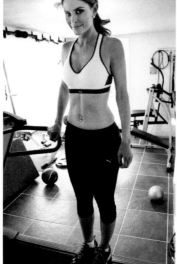

Step-Up and Leg Kickback

Stand next to a step or bench; if you have shaky balance, place it near something you can hold onto throughout the movement. Step up with your left foot.

Step up with your right foot so that both feet are on the steps.

Keeping both legs straight, kick your left leg back behind you as high as you can comfortably go. Return your foot to the original position.

Repeat kickback on the other side. Step back down. Do a total of 10 step-ups and 10 kickbacks on each leg. Talk about a butt burner!

TARGET ZONE **THIGHS**

BONUS ZONE **BUTT**

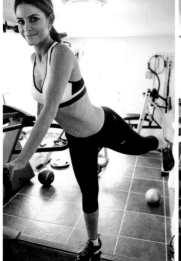
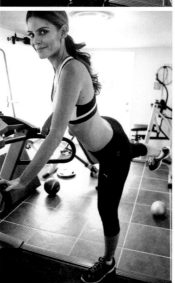

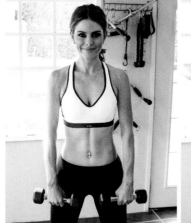
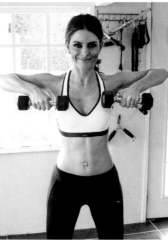

Upright Rows

Stand holding a dumbbell in each hand with your palms facing behind you, at about thigh height.

Keeping your back straight, lift the weights and point your elbows out so your upper arms are parallel to the floor. Your palms should still be facing you. Return to the start position. Do 15 reps.

TARGET ZONE **SHOULDERS**

BONUS ZONE **BACK**

WORKOUT CONTINUED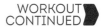

Original EveryGirl Workout

(continued from previous page)

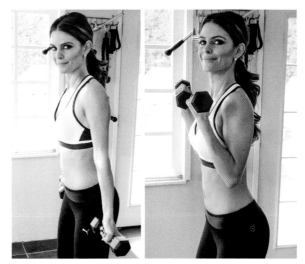

Biceps Curl

Stand holding dumbbells at your sides with your palms facing frontward.

Without moving your upper arms, curl the dumbbells up until they are almost touching your shoulders. Complete 15 reps.

TARGET ZONE BICEPS

BONUS ZONE CORE

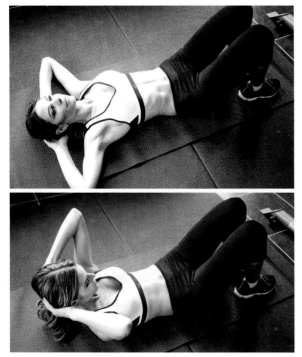

Abdominal Curl

Lie on the ground with your knees bent and your hands lightly placed on the back of your head.

Using your abs, lift your upper body off the ground an inch or two. Do not tug on your head with your hands—these are not situps! Your hands are there only for a little support and to take some pressure off your neck. Complete 50 repetitions.

TARGET ZONE ABS

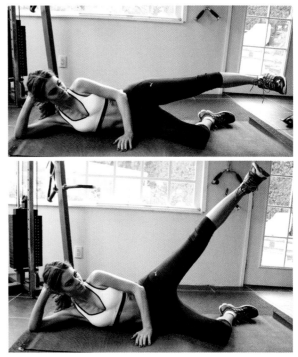

Straight Leg Lift

Lie on your right side with your right knee on the ground and knee bent. Raise your left leg, keeping it straight so that it's not touching your right leg. Rest your head in your right hand, and keep your left hand in front of you on the floor.

Lift your left leg as high as it can go, keeping your foot flexed and toe pointed forward. Complete 15 reps on each side.

TARGET ZONE BUTT

BONUS ZONE ABS

The Medicine Ball Workout

The medicine ball is one of my favorite pieces of exercise equipment because it is versatile, provides some resistance, and can be fun, too. While it's not convenient for travel the way resistance bands are, it's surely a great piece of equipment for home use. Best of all, one ball is all you need to get in a fast and effective total-body workout. Repeat circuit two or three times.

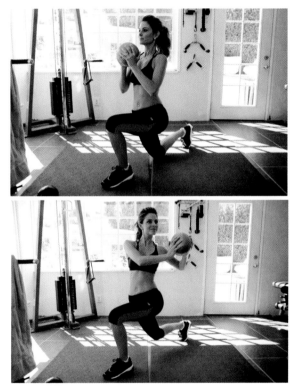

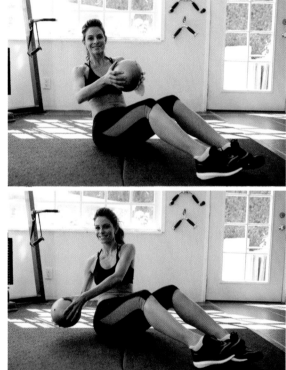

Lunge and Twist

Stand with your feet shoulder-width apart and hold the ball at arm's length in front of your chest. Lunge forward with your left leg so that your thigh is parallel to the ground (and not extending past your toes). Your right knee should almost touch the ground. From there, twist your torso to your left so that you feel a stretch in your right hip, then lunge and twist to the opposite side. Complete 10 controlled reps on each side.

TARGET ZONE THIGHS

BONUS ZONE ABS

Russian Twist

Sit with your butt on the ground with your knees bent and hold the ball at chest level. Lean back slightly. Twist to the right and touch the ball to the ground, then twist all the way back to the left and touch the ball to the ground. Do 10 twists to each side. Advanced: Raise your feet off the ground.

TARGET ZONE ABS

BONUS ZONE LOWER BACK

WORKOUT CONTINUED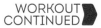

The Medicine Ball Workout

(continued from previous page)

Squat and Press

Hold the ball at chest level. With your feet shoulder-width apart, squat down so that your thighs are parallel to the floor (and make sure your knees don't extend past your toes). As you stand up, press the ball straight overhead. Lower the ball to chest level and begin the next rep. Do 15 reps. Advanced: Do the movement on one leg, 10 on each side.

TARGET ZONE THIGHS

BONUS ZONE SHOULDERS

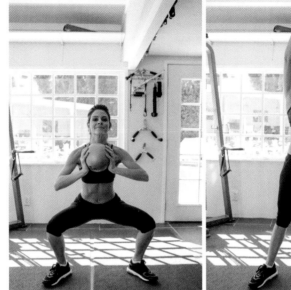
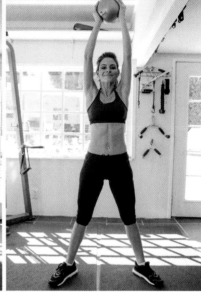

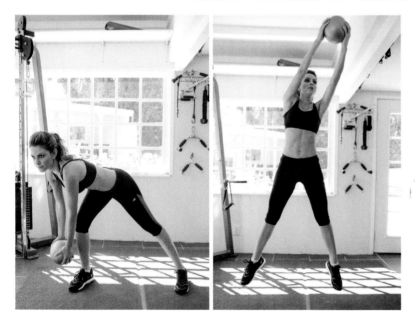

Medicine Ball Chop

Stand with your feet about shoulder-width apart and hold the medicine ball in front of you with both hands. Lower the ball to your right foot by bending your right knee but keeping your left leg straight—this will feel a little like a combination of a squat and a lunge. Rise up and drive the ball toward the ceiling over your left shoulder, coming off your toes as if you were going to throw the ball (but don't throw it!). Return to the starting position and repeat on the other side. You should be holding the ball with both hands at all times. When done fluidly, it looks like a chopping movement. Do 20 reps, 10 on each side. I love this total-body move—it works your upper body, lower body, and core.

TARGET ZONE ABS

BONUS ZONE SHOULDERS

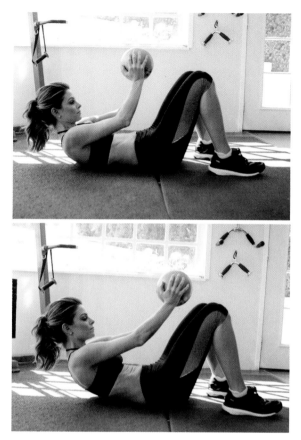

Ball Crunch-Up

Lie flat on the ground holding the ball straight up so that your arms are at a 90-degree angle to your body. Without moving the position of your arms (keep the ball pointed toward the ceiling), crunch up slightly, lifting your shoulders off the ground. Do 20 reps..

TARGET ZONE ABS

BONUS ZONE SHOULDERS

My Favorite Ab Exercises

→ 50 sit-ups: 20 straight up and down; 10 to each side, with one ankle crossed over the opposite knee; and then 10 straight up and down again.

→ Medicine ball crunch-ups with a friend. Throwing the ball back and forth to your workout partner makes it feel more like a game and less like a workout.

→ Contracting my abs throughout the day; on the set, in the car, while waiting in line at the store, there's always time for an ab workout.

The Door-Gym Workout

This wall unit cable system that attaches to your door can help you do several moves that will work your body. It's especially good if you want a gym-quality cable system. At worst you can opt for a resistance band and stimulate the same muscle groups.

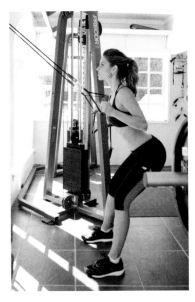

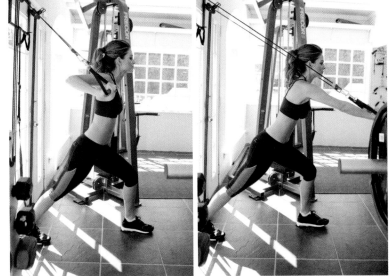

Standing Cable Row

Stand with feet shoulder-width apart, knees soft and slightly bent, arms straight on handles. Draw elbows back until shoulder blades are pulled together, maintain elbows at a 90 degree angle, slowly return hands to start position. Repeat 20 times using a minimum of 25 lbs.

TARGET ZONE LOWER BACK

BONUS ZONES BICEPS AND ABS

Standing Wall Cable Fly

With legs staggered, grasp handles and place hands at shoulder height, elbows at 90 degrees, soft knees, slight hinge forward away from door. Press both hands forward in front of chest, then return to start position. Repeat 20 times.

TARGET ZONE CHEST

BONUS ZONES SHOULDERS AND TRICEPS

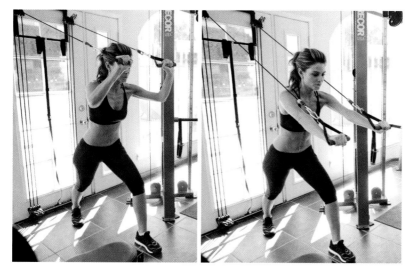

Triceps Cable Extension

Stand facing away from anchor point in a staggered stance, hips hinged slightly forward. Hold handles with palms facing down, arms bent 90 degrees and hands a few inches from your face. Keep upper arms stable and straighten elbows using your triceps for movement. Repeat 20 times.

TARGET ZONE TRICEPS

BONUS ZONES SHOULDERS AND ABS

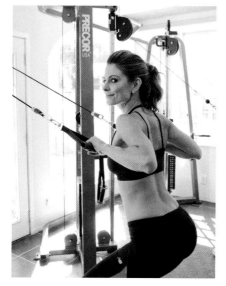

Cable Row

Stand far enough away to generate tension in the cable, arms straight, and sit into a squat position. Pull both arms back in a row. Repeat 20 times.

TARGET ZONE BACK

BONUS ZONES ARMS AND ABS

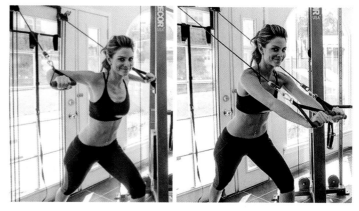

Chest Press

Stand tall with back toward the anchor. Stagger stance one foot in front of other for stability, holding handles palm facing down, elbows lifted to shoulder height. Press your hands forward until they are in front of your chest, then return elbows back to sides. Repeat 20 times.

TARGET ZONE CHEST

BONUS ZONE SHOULDERS

The Door-Gym Workout
(continued from previous page)

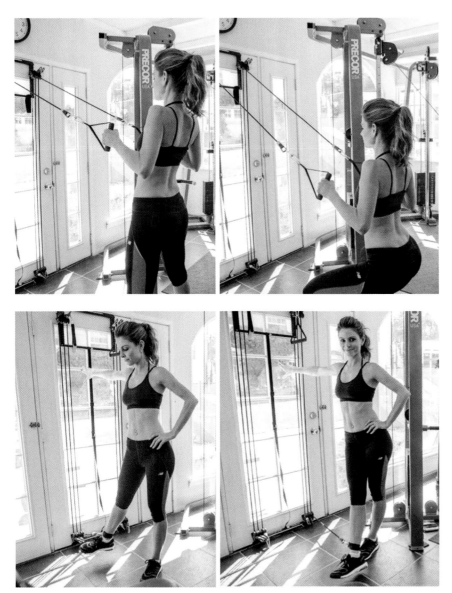

Standing Squat

Stand tall, with feet-shoulder width apart, chest lifted, and elbows bent 90 degrees at your sides.

Maintain the row while you drive your hips back placing weight in heels to just under 90 degree angle at the knee. Drive through your heels and squat back to start position. Repeat 20 times.

TARGET ZONES BUTT AND THIGHS

BONUS ZONES BACK AND POSTURE

Inner-Thigh Cable Pull

Anchoring the ankle to the cable holding wall or bar for balance, stand on non anchored leg with chest lifted and posture tall.

Draw the weighted leg across the midline of the body using the inner thigh to pull. Return the leg to start position using the thigh. Repeat 20 times.

TARGET ZONE INNER THIGHS

BONUS ZONES BUTT AND BALANCE

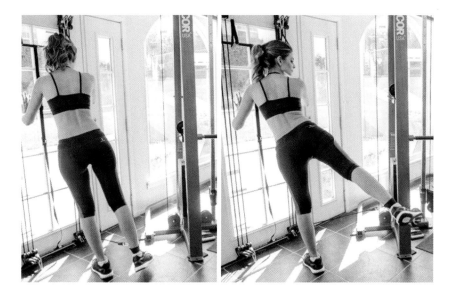

Leg Extension

Anchor cable around one leg, bracing your body with the other leg.

Abs tight, slight hinge of the hops forward, lift the weighted leg behind you using the glute to give height. Return to start position. Repeat 20 times.

TARGET ZONES CALVES AND THIGHS

BONUS ZONES BUTT AND BALANCE

Dumbbell/Hand Weight Workout

Like the medicine ball, a pair of dumbbells is also extremely versatile. There are so many moves you can do to challenge your muscles, burn calories, and keep yourself fit. Don't make the mistake of going too light. You want a weight that's challenging, but not so heavy that you can't maintain proper form. I like to use 5- to 15-pound weights, depending on the exercise. As a general guideline, start with a medium weight and if they're too light or too heavy for certain exercises, you can just adjust the weight or the number of times you perform the exercise to create the best challenge. Repeat this circuit two or three times.

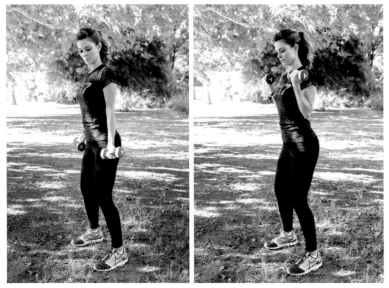

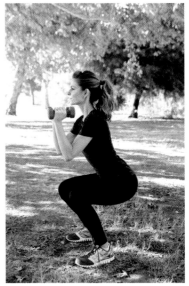

Curl

Hold the dumbbells at your sides, then curl them up to your shoulders. You can do both at the same time or alternate your arms. Do 12 on each side.

TARGET ZONE BICEPS   BONUS ZONE BACK

Slow Squat

Hold the dumbbells to your sides and stand with your feet shoulder-width apart. Take 4 or 5 seconds to squat down and 4 or 5 seconds to stand back up—doing it slowly is the key here! Aim for 8 reps.

TARGET ZONE THIGHS

BONUS ZONE BUTT

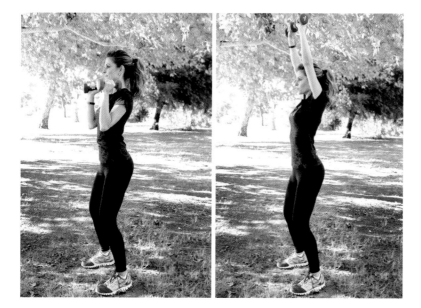

Overhead Press

Stand upright with your feet shoulder-width apart, elbows bent, dumbbells at shoulder height. Press both of the weights over your head to form a letter Y (instead of straight up). Slowly control the lowering of the elbows back to starting position. Do 15 reps.

TARGET ZONE SHOULDERS   BONUS ZONE BACK

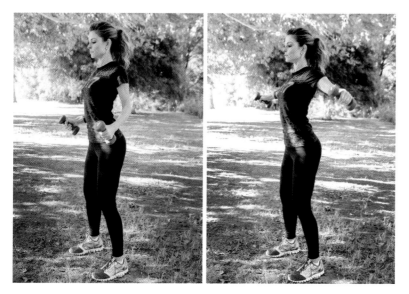

Standing Lateral Fly

Stand upright, feet shoulder-width apart, arms in the Barbie stance. Raise your arms 90 degrees out and up to shoulder height. Control the descent back to the starting position.

TARGET ZONE SHOULDERS   BONUS ZONE BACK

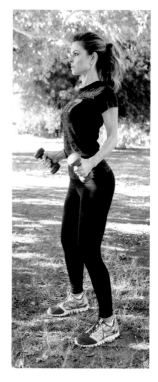

WHAT IS THE BARBIE STANCE?

The Barbie stance is for good posture. Stand with your shoulders down and back, chest up, elbows slightly bent . . . like a Barbie doll!

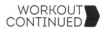

WORKOUT CONTINUED

The Dumbbell Workout
(continued from previous page)

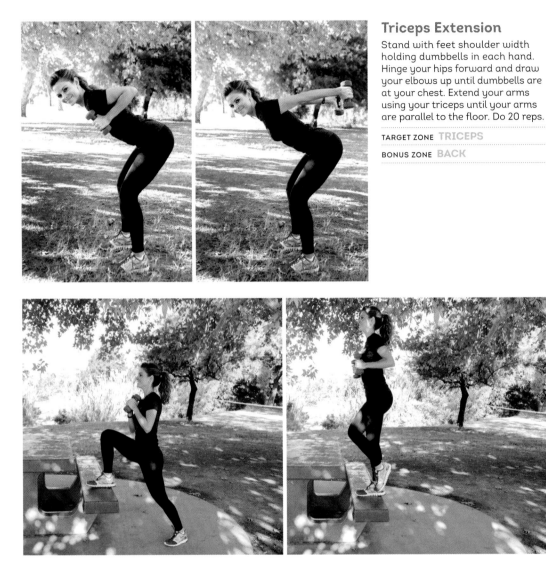

Triceps Extension

Stand with feet shoulder width holding dumbbells in each hand. Hinge your hips forward and draw your elbows up until dumbbells are at your chest. Extend your arms using your triceps until your arms are parallel to the floor. Do 20 reps.

TARGET ZONE TRICEPS

BONUS ZONE BACK

Dumbbell Step-Up

Holding the dumbbells in front of your chest, take a step onto a stair or a stable bench. Bring your second leg up, then step down. Do 12 reps on each leg. Advanced: Press the dumbbells over your head as you step up.

TARGET ZONE BUTT   BONUS ZONE THIGHS

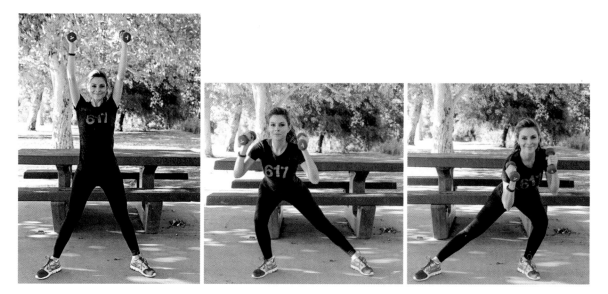

Overhead Lateral Lunge

Stand upright, feet shoulder-width apart, holding dumbbells overhead with arms extended. Lunge to one side, planting your foot facing forward. Your trailing leg will be extended and you'll feel a stretch in the inner thigh. Step back to the starting position and repeat on the opposite leg. Do 10 reps on each side.

TARGET ZONE THIGHS   BONUS ZONES SHOULDER AND BUTT.

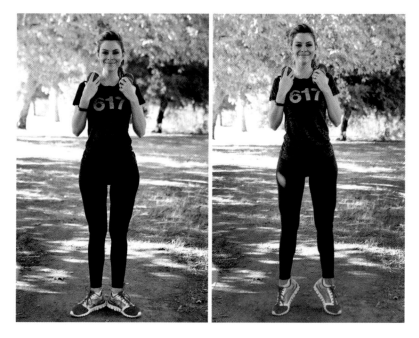

Standing Ballet Calf Raise

Start in first position, heels together and toes turned out, dumbbells close to your sides or at your shoulders. Pressing through your toes, rise as high as you can using your calves to lift, then lower. Complete 20 reps. Repeat the circuit 3 or 4 times.

TARGET ZONE CALVES

BONUS ZONE ANKLES

Andrea's Urban Workout

Andrea Orbeck is an amazing athlete, personal trainer to the stars, and a close friend. She's shared with me workout circuits that can be easily integrated into your everyday life, from the front yard to the park, and you can take these exercises with you anywhere. It's a great way to get outside and easily make exercise a part of your daily routine. Do 10-12 reps of each move.

FULL-BODY Park Bench Workout Series

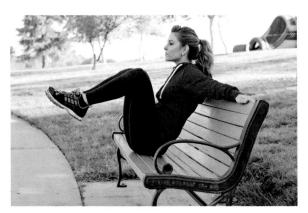

Jackknife

Balance on your tailbone with your hands at your sides for stability and balance. Leaning back slightly, pull your knees to your chest and use your abs to extend your feet forward. Hold for 30 seconds, keeping your abs tight.

TARGET ZONE ABS

GET CREATIVE, FIND A TREE OR OTHER MARKER NEAR A PARK BENCH AND SPRINT, LUNGE, AND SIDESTEP BETWEEN THE TWO.

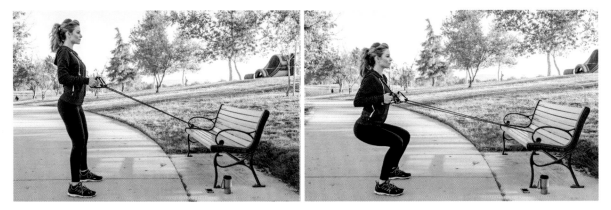

Bench Band Squats

Maintain your elbows in the row position. Using your glutes and quads, drive your hips back and down below your knees. Rise back to standing position, pressing the weight through your heels. Complete 20 reps.

TARGET ZONE BUTT   BONUS ZONE THIGHS

Bench Squats

Stand tall, one foot away from the seat and arms extended for balance. Lower your hips toward the seat. Just before you touch, return slowly to standing position, pushing through the heels and squeezing your glutes to drive your hips forward.

TARGET ZONE THIGHS

BONUS ZONE BUTT

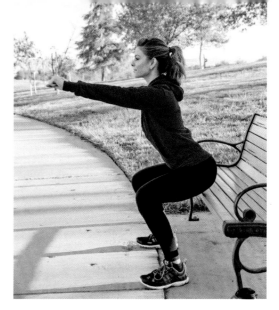

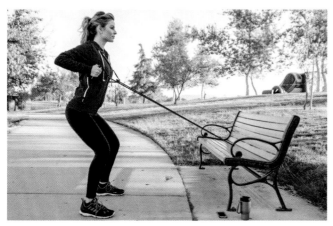

Standing Bench Row

Anchor the resistance band to a sturdy object. Hold the ends of the band in each hand and stand far enough away from the anchor point to generate tension in the band. With arms straight, pull both arms back in a row. Complete 20 reps.

TARGET ZONE BACK

BONUS ZONE ABS

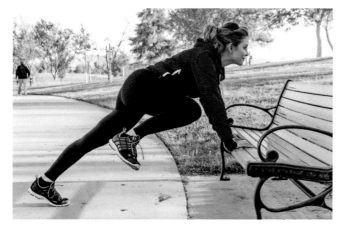

Bench Mountain Climber

Start in plank, hands on a chair with legs extended and weight on your toes. Alternate lifting one knee along the body, toward the shoulder, return leg to start and repeat with other leg. Complete 20 reps (10 on each leg).

TARGET ZONE ABS

BONUS ZONE SHOULDERS

WORKOUT CONTINUED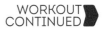

Andrea's Urban Workout
(continued from previous page)

Burpee

Start in plank with your hands on the bench. Jump feet forward to a crouched position. Then explode into the air with hands over your head.
Return hands to bench and jump hands back to plank. Complete 10 reps.

TARGET ZONES THIGHS AND ABS   **BONUS ZONE** HEART

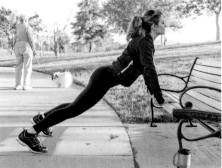
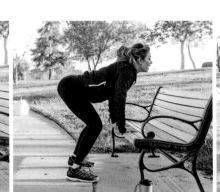

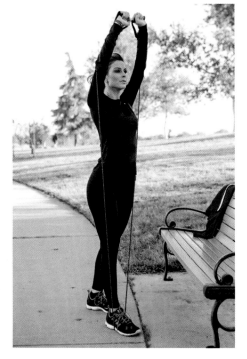

Standing Band Overhead Press

With a staggered stance, anchor the resistance band under your front foot. With the handles at your shoulders, push your hands overhead until your elbows are straight, then return your elbows back down. Complete 20 reps.

TARGET ZONE SHOULDERS

BONUS ZONE BACK

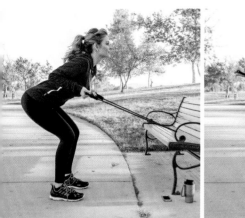
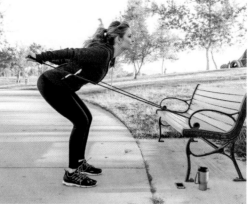

Bench Triceps Extension with Resistance Band

Stand with your elbows at your sides, knees unlocked, and bend over at the waist. Bend and straighten your elbows at your sides using your triceps for movement. Complete 15 reps.

TARGET ZONE TRICEPS

BONUS ZONE BACK

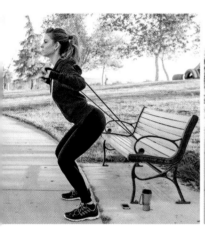
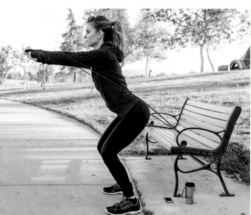

Standing Band Chest Fly

Anchor the resistance band to a fixed surface. Keep your hands at shoulder height, elbows bent at a 90-degree angle, knees soft, frame bent slightly forward. Press both hands forward in front of your chest and return to start position. Complete 20 reps.

TARGET ZONE CHEST

BONUS ZONE SHOULDERS

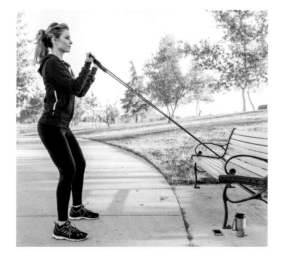

Standing Bench Biceps Curl

Stand upright with your knees unlocked and your palms facing up. Stand back far enough to generate tension in the resistance band while keeping your elbows elevated. Bend your elbows to a biceps curl. Complete 15 reps.

TARGET ZONE BICEPS

BONUS ZONE BACK

WORKOUT CONTINUED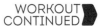

Andrea's Urban Workout
(continued from previous page)

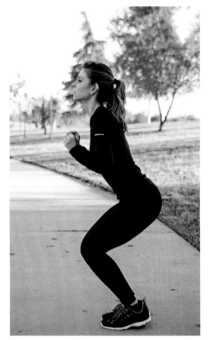

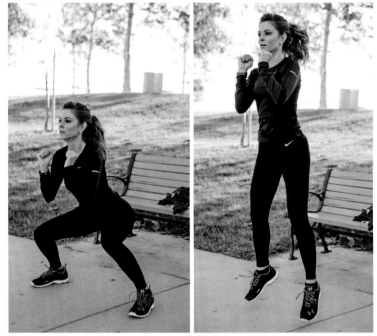

Lateral Shuffle

Lateral shuffles are a great way to engage your outer glutes and to track your knees correctly. Push off with your lead leg and stay low in your form to isolate your butt and quads. Complete 20 reps in each direction.

TARGET ZONES THIGHS AND BUTT

Plyometrics

Plyos are a great way to generate strength, muscle tone, and power in a short period of time. Start in a low squat position. Generating power through the legs, explode out of the squat and then land softly back into the squat with your knees soft to absorb the impact. Repeat 15 times.

TARGET ZONE THIGHS

BONUS ZONES BUTT AND HEART

POOR FORM

Form is important for a squat to target the correct muscle groups and to avoid straining the knee. Proper form is avoiding the knee traveling over the toes, as seen here.

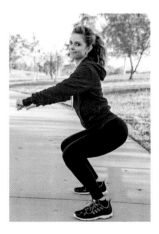

316

FULL-BODY Tree Workout Series

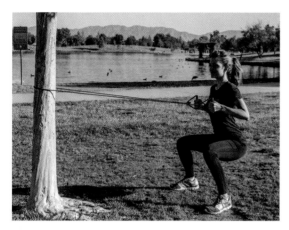

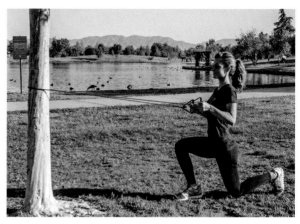

Band Squat

Wrap the resistance band securely around the trunk of the tree with your elbows in a row position. Lower your hips under knee level. Drive your hips back to a standing position, pressing up through your heels. Complete 15 reps.

TARGET ZONE THIGHS   BONUS ZONE BUTT

Alternating Reverse Lunge

Wrap the resistance band securely around the tree. Stand upright with your feet shoulder-width apart and step backward with one leg into a lunge position, using the front leg for control. Return to start position. Repeat 15 times per leg.

TARGET ZONE: THIGHS   BONUS ZONE BUTT

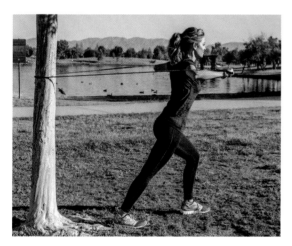

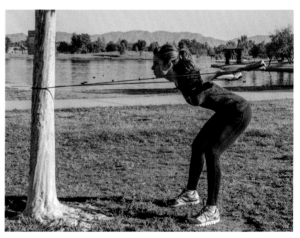

Chest Press

Stand with hands at shoulder height and elbows at a 90-degree angle with knees unlocked, legs staggered. Press both hands forward in front of your chest and then return to start position. Complete 20 reps.

TARGET ZONE CHEST

BONUS ZONE SHOULDERS

Triceps Extension

Stand with your elbows at your sides, knees unlocked, bend over at the hips. Using the triceps for movement, bend and straighten your elbows at your sides. Complete 15 reps.

TARGET ZONE TRICEPS   BONUS ZONE SHOULDERS

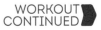

WORKOUT CONTINUED

Andrea's Urban Workout
(continued from previous page)

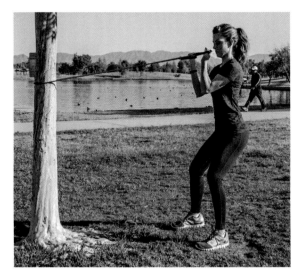

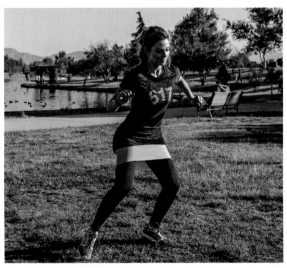

Biceps Curl

Wrap resistance band around the tree and stand in an athletic stance, far enough away from the tree so the band has tension, arms straight in front of you. Curl both hands toward your chin simultaneously. Complete 15 reps.

TARGET ZONE BICEPS

BONUS ZONE UPPER BACK

Side Shuffle

Push off with your lead leg and stay low in your form to isolate your butt and quads. Add the band for more resistance. Complete 20 reps in each direction.

TARGET ZONES THIGHS AND BUTT

BONUS ZONE INNER THIGH

Freestanding Hip Extension Using Hipster or Thera-Band

Standing straight with the band across your hips, extend the resisted leg back as far as you can while keeping the knee straight. Then return the leg to the starting position. Complete 20 reps on each leg.

TARGET ZONE BUTT

BONUS ZONE THIGHS

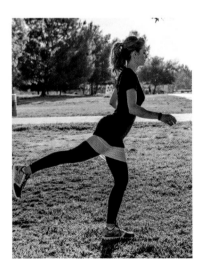

318

Abduction/Side Leg Raise Using Hipster or Thera-Band

Standing with hipster wrapped around your thighs, knees bent and holding a surface for balance, lift one leg along the side of your body as high as you can and slowly return to start position. Focus on lifting with your glutes. Complete 30 reps per side.

TARGET ZONE BUTT

BONUS ZONE BALANCE

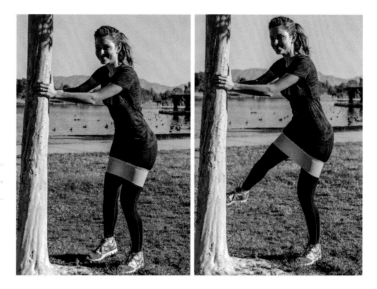

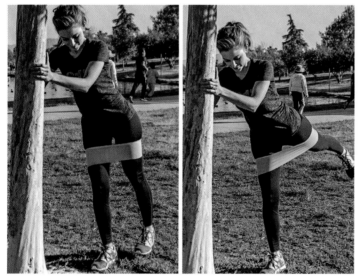

Hip Extension Using Hipster or Thera-Band

Standing secure with the band across your hips, balance on one leg and extend the other leg straight behind you, resisting the band and using the glutes to get leg height. Complete 20 reps on each leg.

TARGET ZONE BUTT

BONUS ZONE LOWER BACK

Q You've trained Victoria Secret models before and after they've had babies. You've also trained EveryGirls. How are the two groups of women similar?

Their physiology. If you eat more than your body's caloric requirements, those calories can be stored as fat. If you are lazy and don't do resistance training, you will have flat and soft muscles. A model's legs may be long, but you can't use them to outrun a slow metabolism.

Q What is your philosophy on weight loss?

We should be more concerned with the loss of excessive fat versus weight. Too often, people step on the scale and rest their hopes and self-esteem on a numerical value between their toes. A victory or defeat of two to three pounds on the scale could easily be water, digesting food, and the weight of a poop. Focus on how lean you are, your body fat levels, and the girth of your body.

Q What's the one change you've made in your fitness routine that's really made a difference in how you look or feel?

Intensity is key. Out with the old theory of long, boring, and steady-state cardio! In with the fat-incinerating benefits of high-intensity interval training (HIIT)!

Q How do you stay motivated to eat right and exercise?

I use clothes that I love and look good on me when I'm leaner, I use events on the calendar that I am excited about—however small—and I use how I feel when I literally wake up in the morning. When I am rested, feel strong and sexy, and get that workout high, I credit good, healthy choices.

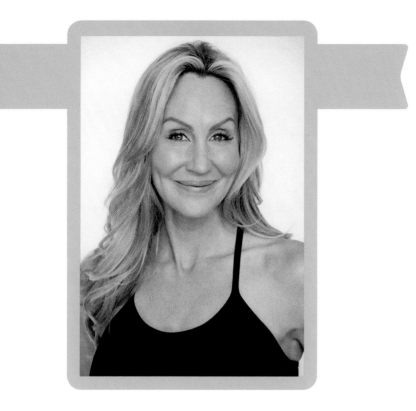

Q **How do you deal with the guilt when you've eaten something you "shouldn't" be eating or you miss a workout?**

I never feel guilty about food or exercise. I accept that it's a part of the entire day's schedule and sometimes cannot be done. When my schedule is jam-packed and there is simply no time to exercise, I watch my caloric intake to balance it out.

Q **What's your advice for someone struggling to lose weight?**

Patience and science. Look away from the BS infomercial promising instant change and give yourself the real time it takes to accomplish goals. Learn and understand that looking and feeling your best happens over time with consistency, activity, and healthy eating.

Acknowledgments

I have so many people to thank for helping put this book together. First let me thank my parents. My parents, Costas and Litsa, who inspire me in so many ways. Thank you to my colleagues who contributed their expertise toward making this the best it could be: My dear friend Andrea Orbeck. Andrea, your in-depth of knowledge of exercise, diet, nutrition, fitness and anatomy, matched with your sensitivity, passion, and giving nature make you the rarest of trainers and rarest of people. I'm so thankful for all you contributed to help my readers and am so blessed to have you in my life. Thank you to my dear friend Yogi Cameron Alborzian for saving me and my loved ones so many times and for all the valuable lessons you have taught me. Thank you for taking me on this incredible health journey and for all the laughs along the way. Dave Zinczenko, Steve Perrine, George Karabotsos, Kimberly Miller, Mike Smith, and the team at Galvanized Media, thank you for believing in this book; and Marnie Cochran, Nina Shield, Jennifer Garza, and the team at Random House for publishing it. Ted Spiker, I know I probably bored you with all the fact-checking—but thank you for everything! Thank you to my teams at WME—Jon Rosen and especially Andy McNichol for all you did to help make this book come to life. Gary Mantoosh, Brett Ruttenburg, and Jami Kandel at BWR—guys, I love you, and thank you for all your tireless work to promote this book—as well as my family at Morris/Yorn, Kevin Yorn, Nick Gladden, Logan Clare, and Melodie Moore for all you do for me. Elise Donoghue, your beautiful photos pop off the page and make these books real for people; thank you for always being so on board for anything and everything. And Stephen Lemieux for additional

THE EVERYGIRL'S GUIDE TO DIET AND FITNESS

photography—thanks for coming off the bench when we needed you. Michael Simon of Startraks, thank you for always being so generous with your photo galleries; I really appreciate it. An extra-special thank you to my staff, Pat Lambert and Christa Lenk, without you guys nothing is ever possible. Pat, a huge shout-out for helping shoulder so much of this with me, can't thank you enough.

I'd also like to thank my friends who have supported and contributed to this book: Angie Harmon, Bethenny Frankel, Kim and Khloe Kardashian, Giada De Laurentiis, Jessica Alba, Jane Seymour, Suzanne Somers, Karina Smirnoff, Rebecca Romijn, Stacy Kiebler, Serena Williams, Mario Lopez, Derek Hough, Perez Hilton, Betty Wong, Lucy Danziger, Michele Promaulayko, and Tara Kraft. Your willingness to take the time out of your busy schedules to share your knowledge with the EveryGirls out there and to support me, brought me to tears. I'm so incredibly thankful for all your love and support and hope that I can always be even more supportive of all of you!

Keven, without you, there is no book. Thank you for helping me craft a series of books that help women everywhere figure things out when most don't have the time or money! You are so talented, and I'm the luckiest girl in the world to have you.

And thank you, the EveryGirl reader and supporter, for being part of this adventure. I was once really lost on how to find success in areas of life, diet and fitness notwithstanding. I figured

323

things out, eventually, as I hope you do, but I have learned that the journey never ends. When I wrote my first book I didn't know it would connect with you the way it did. Having "been there," I was genuinely just sharing what I do to make my life easier and better in order to help. I wrote this latest version for the same reason and because you taught me to realize that my journey is your journey. Every time I meet one of you and you've shared your passions, ideas, and advice in return, it makes me smile. I ended my last book saying I believe at the end of the day we are all truly on this planet merely to help one another—and I still believe that. So lets keep helping each other.

I hope you benefit greatly from *The EveryGirl's Guide to Diet and Fitness* and get fit and healthy. But I also pray, in so doing, that you will consider how you as an EveryGirl treat yourself and others. We need to love ourselves more, accept our flaws, and accept that it takes time to work on them; as well as be empathetic, helpful, and kind to others. And we should try not to be jealous. Jealousy prevents YOU from moving forward. We need to work more to lift each other up, rather than tear each other down. Be supportive of one another not competitive.

As far as weight loss goes, it took me years to find my way on the journey. As Oprah says, I needed to finally have that "aha" moment. Whether you get that moment through this book or another, when the time is right and you are ready, you will lose the weight. Just be patient and don't get discouraged.

And remember, they never show anyone's flaws in magazines, but we all have them! The difference between you and me is a glam squad, great lighting, and photo retouching.

As I said, tweet me any questions you may have. Or e-mail me at theeverygirlsguide@gmail.com, which is easier to keep track of. I genuinely want to help and will do my best to answer all your questions.

And please, don't ever hesitate to stop me and share your thoughts on the books and what subjects you'd like to see more of. I hope you benefit from the *EveryGirl's Guide to Diet and Fitness,* and I hope to see and hear from you soon.

All My Love,
Maria

My Social Media Accounts:

TWITTER: @MARIAMENOUNOS

INSTAGRAM: @MARIAMENOUNOS

FACEBOOK: FACEBOOK.COM/MARIAMENOUNOS

About the Authors

MARIA MENOUNOS is a host, reporter, television personality, filmmaker, producer, actor, and *New York Times* bestselling author of *The EveryGirl's Guide to Life*. The host of *Extra* since 2011, her acting credits include *One Tree Hill, Entourage, Scrubs, The Mindy Project, Kickin' It Old Skool, Tropic Thunder,* and *Fantastic Four*. She was a semi-finalist on *Dancing with the Stars* and is a semi-professional wrestler with the World Wrestling Federation. She's the CEO of AfterBuzzTV.com and BlackHollywoodLive.com and the executive producer and star of the Oxygen series *Chasing Maria Menounos*.

KEVEN UNDERGARO is a producer, filmmaker, entrepreneur, and co-author of *The EveryGirl's Guide to Life* with longtime partner, Maria Menounos. He is the creator of the online broadcast networks AfterBuzzTV.com and BlackHollywoodLive.com and executive producer of Oxygen's *Chasing Maria Menounos*.